SUBSTANCE ABUSE ASSESSMENT, INTERVENTIONS AND TREATMENT

AMERICA'S SUBSTANCE ABUSE AND MENTAL HEALTH WORKFORCE

ISSUES AND NEEDS

SUBSTANCE ABUSE ASSESSMENT, INTERVENTIONS AND TREATMENT

Additional books in this series can be found on Nova's website under the Series tab.

Additional E-books in this series can be found on Nova's website under the E-book tab.

MENTAL ILLNESSES AND TREATMENTS

Additional books in this series can be found on Nova's website under the Series tab.

Additional E-books in this series can be found on Nova's website under the E-book tab.

SUBSTANCE ABUSE ASSESSMENT, INTERVENTIONS AND TREATMENT

AMERICA'S SUBSTANCE ABUSE AND MENTAL HEALTH WORKFORCE

ISSUES AND NEEDS

OMRI GALINSKY
EDITOR

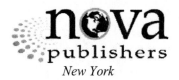

publishers
New York

Copyright © 2013 by Nova Science Publishers, Inc.

All rights reserved. No part of this book may be reproduced, stored in a retrieval system or transmitted in any form or by any means: electronic, electrostatic, magnetic, tape, mechanical photocopying, recording or otherwise without the written permission of the Publisher.

For permission to use material from this book please contact us:
Telephone 631-231-7269; Fax 631-231-8175
Web Site: http://www.novapublishers.com

NOTICE TO THE READER

The Publisher has taken reasonable care in the preparation of this book, but makes no expressed or implied warranty of any kind and assumes no responsibility for any errors or omissions. No liability is assumed for incidental or consequential damages in connection with or arising out of information contained in this book. The Publisher shall not be liable for any special, consequential, or exemplary damages resulting, in whole or in part, from the readers' use of, or reliance upon, this material. Any parts of this book based on government reports are so indicated and copyright is claimed for those parts to the extent applicable to compilations of such works.

Independent verification should be sought for any data, advice or recommendations contained in this book. In addition, no responsibility is assumed by the publisher for any injury and/or damage to persons or property arising from any methods, products, instructions, ideas or otherwise contained in this publication.

This publication is designed to provide accurate and authoritative information with regard to the subject matter covered herein. It is sold with the clear understanding that the Publisher is not engaged in rendering legal or any other professional services. If legal or any other expert assistance is required, the services of a competent person should be sought. FROM A DECLARATION OF PARTICIPANTS JOINTLY ADOPTED BY A COMMITTEE OF THE AMERICAN BAR ASSOCIATION AND A COMMITTEE OF PUBLISHERS.

Additional color graphics may be available in the e-book version of this book.

Library of Congress Cataloging-in-Publication Data

ISBN: 978-1-62808-634-8

Published by Nova Science Publishers, Inc. † New York

CONTENTS

Preface		vii
Chapter 1	Report to Congress on the Nation's Substance Abuse and Mental Health Workforce Issues *Substance Abuse and Mental Health Services Administration*	1
Chapter 2	Report to Congress: Addictions Treatment Workforce Development *Substance Abuse and Mental Health Services Administration*	79
Index		133

PREFACE

The Substance Abuse and Mental Health Services Administration (SAMHSA) has prepared these reports to Congress to provide an overview of the facts and issues affecting the substance abuse and mental health workforce in America. SAMHSA's reports cover the behavioral health workforce in its entirety because many data sources and programs report by profession or discipline rather than population served (e.g., social workers, psychologists, and counselors), whether providing prevention services or treatment and whether serving persons with substance use disorders, mental health conditions, or both. Data specific to the substance use disorder treatment workforce will be provided wherever available. This book also includes demographic data as well as a discussion of key issues and challenges such as staff turnover, aging of the workforce, inadequate compensation, worker shortages, licensing and credentialing issues, and recruitment, and retention and distribution of the workforce. The misunderstandings and often inaccurate perceptions of society about mental illness and addiction as these relate to workforce challenges are also discussed.

Chapter 1 - SAMHSA has prepared this report to Congress to provide an overview of the facts and issues affecting the substance abuse and mental health workforce in America. SAMHSA's report will cover the behavioral health workforce in its entirety because many data sources and programs report by profession or discipline rather than population served (e.g., social workers, psychologists, and counselors), whether providing prevention services or treatment and whether serving persons with substance use disorders, mental health conditions, or both. Data specific to the substance use disorder treatment workforce will be provided wherever available. This report also will include demographic data as well as a discussion of key issues and challenges such as staff turnover, aging of the workforce, inadequate compensation, worker shortages, licensing and credentialing issues, and recruitment, retention and distribution of the workforce. The misunderstandings and often inaccurate perceptions of society about mental illness and addiction as these relate to workforce challenges are also discussed.

Chapter 2 - In 2004, over 23 million Americans age 12 and older needed specialty treatment for alcohol or illicit drug problems (NSDUH, 2005). The human, social and economic costs of not treating substance use disorders are indisputable. Yet, substance use disorders treatment systems are constrained by an inadequate infrastructure to support current and future demands for treatment. The addictions treatment field is facing a workforce crisis. Worker shortages, inadequate compensation, insufficient professional development and stigma currently challenge the field. Increasingly, treatment and recovery support providers also struggle with issues related to recruitment, retention and professional development of staff. The ability to provide quality addictions treatment and recovery support services is severely hampered by these conditions.

In its report on the Fiscal Year (FY) 2006 budget for the Department of Health and Human Services (DHHS), the House Committee on Appropriations stated the following:

> The Committee has concerns that people who are seeking substance abuse treatment are unable to access services due to the lack of an adequate clinical treatment workforce. People seeking treatment often have to wait for weeks or months before they are accepted into a treatment facility. The Committee requests that SAMHSA issue a report, after consultation with stakeholders and other Federal partners, on workforce development for substance abuse treatment professionals. The report should focus on both the recruitment and retention of counselors and on improving the skills of those already providing services as well as ways in which States can play a role. The Committee requests that this report be transmitted to the House and Senate Committees on Appropriations by March 1, 2006. (House report No. 109-143, page 117)

This report was prepared in response to the Committee request. It summarizes trends in addictions treatment and the challenges that confront the treatment workforce. Importantly, it also articulates the perspectives of stakeholders and Federal partners by presenting a series of recommendations aimed at strengthening the field's professional identity. The recommendations in this report reflect some of the best thinking in the field and are intended to provide momentum for ongoing discussions among stakeholders about specific implementation strategies. The report discusses current trends in funding, staff recruitment and retention, patient characteristics and clinical practice and identifies recommendations in the following six areas: infrastructure; leadership and management; recruitment; education and accreditation; retention; and priorities for further study. This report focuses on all professionals who provide addictions treatment and recovery support services, e.g., addictions counselors, physicians, psychologists, nurses, outreach and intake workers, case managers, social workers, marriage and family therapists, recovery support workers and clergy.

In: America's Substance Abuse ...
Editor: Omri Galinsky

ISBN: 978-1-62808-634-8
© 2013 Nova Science Publishers, Inc.

Chapter 1

REPORT TO CONGRESS ON THE NATION'S SUBSTANCE ABUSE AND MENTAL HEALTH WORKFORCE ISSUES[*]

Substance Abuse and Mental Health Services Administration

ABSTRACT

SAMHSA has prepared this report to Congress to provide an overview of the facts and issues affecting the substance abuse and mental health workforce in America. SAMHSA's report will cover the behavioral health workforce in its entirety because many data sources and programs report by profession or discipline rather than population served (e.g., social workers, psychologists, and counselors), whether providing prevention services or treatment and whether serving persons with substance use disorders, mental health conditions, or both. Data specific to the substance use disorder treatment workforce will be provided wherever available. This report also will include demographic data as well as a discussion of key issues and challenges such as staff turnover, aging of the workforce, inadequate compensation, worker shortages, licensing and credentialing issues, and recruitment, retention and distribution of the workforce. The misunderstandings and often

---

[*] This is an edited, reformatted and augmented version of the Substance Abuse and Mental Health Services Administration, dated January 24, 2013.

inaccurate perceptions of society about mental illness and addiction as these relate to workforce challenges are also discussed.

EXECUTIVE SUMMARY

In its report on the fiscal year (FY) 2012 budget for the Department of Health and Human Services (HHS), the Senate Appropriations Committee Subcommittee on Labor, Health, and Human Services, Education, and Related Agencies (LHHS-ED) requested the Substance Abuse and Mental Health Services Administration (SAMHSA) provide the Committee with a workforce report, specifically addressing the addictions workforce and SAMHSA's collaboration with the Health Resources and Services Administration (HRSA). The Subcommittee language is as follows:

> *Addiction Services Workforce.* – The Committee notes the growing workforce crisis in the addictions field due to high turnover rates, worker shortages, an aging workforce, stigma and inadequate compensation. The Mental Health Parity and Addiction Equity Act and the Patient Protection and Affordable Care Act are anticipated to increase the number of individuals who will seek substance use disorder services and may exacerbate current workforce challenges. As the provision of quality substance use disorder services is dependent on an adequate qualified workforce and SAMHSA is the lead federal agency charged with improving these services, the Committee expects SAMHSA to focus on developing the addiction workforce and identify ways to address the current and future workforce needs of the addiction field. The Committee directs SAMHSA to submit a report by March 31, 2012, on current workforce issues in the addiction field, as well as the status and funding of its substance use disorder services workforce initiatives. This report should also detail how SAMHSA is working with HRSA to address addiction service workforce needs and should identify the two agencies' specific roles, responsibilities, funding streams and action steps aimed at strengthening the addiction services workforce (Senate Report 112-84, page 122).

While the workforce report was requested specifically for the addiction treatment workforce, (including those funded by HRSA's Bureau of Health Professions and the Department of Labor). The information on the behavioral health[1] workforce is drawn from multiple resources as there is no single federal data source at this point in time.

The impact of the Affordable Care Act and the Mental Health Parity and Addiction Equity Act (MHPAEA), which will increase access and alter service settings, is also discussed. The enactment of both of these laws may reshape the workforce and the delivery of services. For example, the Affordable Care Act is moving the field toward the integration of services with primary care, which has significant workforce implications in regard to team approaches and the new roles and responsibilities for staff. Bureau of Labor Statistics (BLS) projections made prior to the passage of MHPAEA and Affordable Care Act already indicated higher than normal growth for a number of behavioral health professions.

This report also describes SAMHSA's efforts to address many of these issues through its current programs and its eight Strategic Initiatives. In addition, the report presents a summary of collaborations between SAMHSA and HRSA, including a jointly sponsored listening session on the behavioral health workforce. HRSA and SAMHSA have worked collaboratively to address behavioral health workforce issues by sharing information about efforts within each agency and by developing, funding, and managing joint projects such as the Center for Integrated Health Solutions (CIHS), the minimum data set (MDS) project, and the training of practitioners about military culture to enhance service provision for veterans and their families. Many of these projects and efforts are described in this report.

SAMHSA is keenly aware that to achieve its mission to reduce the impact of substance abuse and mental illness on America's communities, a well-trained, educated and fully functioning workforce is needed. Likewise, HRSA is aware that to achieve its mission to improve health and achieve health equity through access to quality services, a skilled health workforce and innovative programs, it must address behavioral health as an essential part of the health care landscape in America. SAMHSA and HRSA are working together toward these aims.

INTRODUCTION TO REPORT

An adequate supply of a well-trained workforce is the foundation for an effective service delivery system. Workforce issues, which have been of concern for decades, have taken on a greater sense of urgency with the passage of recent parity and health reform legislation. SAMHSA is fully cognizant of the impact that workforce issues have on the infrastructure of the behavioral health delivery system and services, and seeks to address these issues through a variety of initiatives and programs. SAMHSA also recognizes that increasing the size of the workforce, recruiting a more diverse, younger workforce, and retaining trained and qualified staff are necessary to provide for the behavioral health needs of the nation's population.

In the past decade, SAMHSA commissioned workforce reports to identify major workforce issues and develop recommendations to address these challenges. These reports, *An Action Plan for Behavioral Health Workforce Development* (SAMHSA, 2007), *Report to Congress: Addiction Treatment Workforce Development* (SAMHSA, 2006), and *Strengthening Professional Identity: Challenges of the Addition Treatment Workforce* (SAMHSA, 2006a), led to the continuing support of some existing programs and the development of some new workforce efforts. Behavioral health workforce initiatives focus on technology transfer and training on evidence-based practices, providing resources, supporting knowledge transfer, recruiting a diverse workforce, and integrating primary and behavioral health care.

Since the publication of SAMHSA's workforce reports, there have been a number of changes that increase the need and demand for behavioral health services. The Affordable Care Act will increase the number of people who are eligible for health care coverage through Medicaid and Exchanges and includes parity for services within its covered services. In addition, as screening for mental illness and substance abuse become more commonplace in primary care, more people will be identified as needing services. Furthermore, workforce shortages will be impacted by additional demands that result from: (1) a large number of returning veterans in need of services; and (2) new state re-entry initiatives to reduce prison populations, a large majority of whom have mental or substance use disorders.

Preparing a workforce that can meet the challenges of the 21st century is an essential component of SAMHSA's strategic plan and programs. SAMHSA has embedded workforce elements in each of the eight Strategic Initiatives, as described in its strategic plan document, *"Leading Change: A Plan for SAMHSA's Roles and Actions 2011-2014,"* (SAMHSA, 2011a). Examples of workforce objectives in each of the Strategic Initiatives include:

1. *Prevention of Substance Abuse and Mental Illness*: Educate the behavioral health field about successful interventions, such as screening, brief intervention, and referral to treatment (SBIRT); and develop and implement training around suicide prevention and prescription drug abuse.

2. *Trauma and Justice*: Provide technical assistance and training strategies to develop practitioners skilled in trauma and trauma-related work and systems that have capacity to prevent, identify, intervene and effectively treat people in a trauma-informed approach.
3. *Military Families*: Develop a public health-informed model of psychological health service systems, staffed by a full range of behavioral health practitioners who are well trained in the culture of the military and the military family and the special risks and needs that impact this population, such as Post-Traumatic Stress Disorder (PTSD) and Traumatic Brain Injury (TBI). The role of peer counselors within this model will also be important to its success.
4. *Recovery Support*: Build an understanding of recovery-oriented practices, including incorporating peers into the current workforce to support peer-run services. Emphasize collaborative relationships with children, youth, and families that involve shared decision-making service options.
5. *Health Reform*: Work with partners and stakeholders to develop a new generation of providers, promote innovation of service delivery through primary care and behavioral health care integration, and increase quality and reduce health care costs through health insurance exchanges and the essential and benchmark benefit plans.
6. *Health Information Technology*: Promote the adoption of electronic health records (EHRs) and the use of health information technology (HIT) through SAMHSA's discretionary program and Block Grant technical assistance efforts.
7. *Data, Outcomes and Quality*: Target quality improvement through workshops, intensive training and resources that promote the adoption of evidence-based practices, and activities to advance the delivery of clinical supervision to foster competency development and staff retention.
8. *Public Awareness and Support*: Ensure that the behavioral health workforce has access to information needed to provide successful prevention, treatment, and recovery services.

BACKGROUND

The Institute of Medicine (IOM; 2006) chronicles efforts beginning as early as the 1970s that attempt to deal with some of the workforce issues regarding mental and substance use disorders, but notes that most have not been sustained long enough or been comprehensive enough to remedy the problems. Shortages of qualified workers, recruitment and retention of staff and an aging workforce have long been cited as problems. Lack of workers in rural/frontier areas and the need for a workforce more reflective of the racial and ethnic composition of the U.S. population create additional barriers to accessing care for many. Recruitment and retention efforts are hampered by inadequate compensation, which discourages many from entering or remaining in the field. In addition, the misperceptions and prejudice surrounding mental and substance use disorders and those who experience them are imputed to those who work in the field.

Of additional concern, a new IOM report (2012) notes that the current workforce is unprepared to meet the mental and substance use disorder treatment needs of the rapidly growing population of older adults. The IOM report's data indicate that 5.6 to 8 million older adults, about one in five, have one or more mental health and substance use conditions which compound the care they need. However, there is a dearth of mental health or substance abuse practitioners who are trained to deal with this population.

Pre-service education and continuing education and training of the workforce have been found wanting, as evidenced by the long delays in adoption of evidence-based practices, under- utilization of technology, and lack of skills in critical thinking (SAMHSA, 2007). These education and training deficiencies are even more problematic with the increasing integration of primary care and mental or substance use disorder treatment, and the focus on improving quality of care and outcomes. As noted by the IOM (2003), all health care personnel, including behavioral health clinicians, should be trained "to deliver patient centered care as members of an interdisciplinary team, emphasizing evidence-based practice, quality improvement approaches and informatics."

Data reported in the 2010 and 2011 National Survey on Drug Use and Health (NSDUH) demonstrates the current unmet need for behavioral health services:

- Approximately 21.6 million persons aged 12 or older (8.4 percent of this population) needed treatment for an illicit drug or alcohol use problem.
- Only 2.3 million (10.8 percent) of those who needed treatment received treatment at a specialty facility (SAMHSA, 2012b).

- Approximately 45.9 million adults aged 18 or older (20 percent of adults) in the United States had any mental illness in the past year.
- Approximately 11.1 million adults aged 18 or older (4.9 percent of adults) reported an unmet need for mental health care in the past year including 5.2 million adults aged 18 or older who reported an unmet need for mental health care and did not receive mental health services in the past year.
- Inability to afford care was cited as the most significant barrier to receiving care for mental health services (43.7 percent of those surveyed who needed services); the lack of coverage and cost of services was cited as a significant barrier in seeking substance use disorders services (32.9 percent of those surveyed who needed services for a substance use disorder (SAMHSA, 2011).

As indicated in the NSDUH data above, many individuals who may need behavioral health services do not access them due to lack of health care coverage. However, health reform will significantly reduce this barrier to behavioral health services. It is estimated that approximately 11 million of the individuals who will have access to coverage beginning in 2014 will have mental and/or substance use disorders and will have access to care with the continued implementation of health reform (SAMHSA, 2011). This increase is expected to strain an already thinly stretched workforce.

In the absence of any available standardized survey instrument or national study that provides the needed information, data for this report are taken from a number of sources. There are two SAMHSA sponsored initiatives that will address the paucity of standardized workforce data. SAMHSA and HRSA are working collaboratively on the development of a MDS, starting with the major behavioral health professional disciplines, which may ameliorate the data scarcity problem in the future. In addition, SAMHSA's Addiction Technology Transfer Centers (ATTCs) conducted a national workforce survey on the addiction treatment workforce which was completed at the end of FY 2012.

CHANGING LANDSCAPE: IMPACT ON THE WORKFORCE

In addition to the enactment of parity and health reform legislation, advancements in research, demand for outcomes and quality improvements, and the empowerment of people in recovery are contributing to changes in practice and the workforce. Major changes to the field include the integration of behavioral health and primary care, a push to accelerate the adoption of evidence-based practices, and a model of care that is recovery-oriented, person-centered, integrated, and utilizes multi-disciplinary teams. Behavioral health has moved to a chronic care, public health model to define needed services. This model recognizes the importance of prevention, the primacy of long-term recovery as its key construct, and is shaped by those with lived experience of recovery. This new care model will require a diverse, skilled, and trained workforce that employs a range of workers, including people in recovery, recovery specialists, case workers and highly trained specialists.

Integrated care will reduce medical costs and result in better outcomes. One study showed that individuals with the most serious mental illnesses and co-occurring disorders living in publicly funded inpatient facilities die at age 53, on average (Parks et al., 2006). A more recent study, using a population based representative sample, found that people with mental health disorders died on the average eight years younger than those without mental health disorders and these deaths were largely due to medical causes rather than accidents or suicides (Druss et al., 2011). People with mental and substance use disorders die from treatable medical conditions such as smoking, obesity, high blood pressure and a variety of other medical disorders (Mertens et al., 2003). Untreated mental and substance use disorders not only negatively impact a person's behavioral health but also lead to worse outcomes for co-occurring physical health problems.

Though the co-occurrence of behavioral and other medical conditions is common, individuals with serious behavioral health conditions who lack financial resources are often unable to access quality care, either for their behavioral health conditions or for other health problems. Good behavioral health is associated with better physical health outcomes, improved educational attainment, increased economic participation, and meaningful social relationships. Further, good health is not possible without good behavioral health (Friedli & Parsonage, 2007). Receipt of behavioral health treatment has been shown to decrease medical care costs significantly (Gerson et al., 2001). Thomas (2006) reported savings of $140 per enrollee per month when coordinated care was provided for high-cost, high-risk Medicaid patients with depression. This coordinated care resulted in a 12.9 percent reduction in cost for this population. Unützer et al. (2008) found that providing coordinated depression and primary care for older adults resulted in reduced symptoms of depression in 45 percent of patients and reduced the per patient care cost an average of $3,000 over four years.

Another significant change in health care is the use of SBIRT. As health reform takes effect, SBIRT will become a part of the ongoing prevention activities resulting in the identification of many more people with, or at risk for, depression and substance use disorders. Many individuals who are identified will receive brief interventions or brief treatment, often conducted by health educators, recovery specialists or other types of staff in the primary care system. Those needing more intensive treatment/recovery services would be referred to specialty treatment providers/practitioners.

The behavioral health care workforce is a complex system, comprising many different professionals ranging from psychiatrists to non-degreed workers and para-professionals. The integration of primary and behavioral health care will impact both the behavioral health and the primary care workforce as primary care staff will be expected to have competencies in behavioral health and behavioral health staff will need competencies associated with working in primary care settings. A study done by the National Association of Community Health Centers (NACHC; 2011) found that 43 percent of physicians working in Federally Qualified Health Centers (FQHCs) were interested in training on medication assisted treatments for persons with addictive disorders. Many FQHC staff also indicated interest in training on Motivational Interviewing, Short-term Interventions, Problem-Focused Treatment, SBIRT, PTSD and trauma interventions.

Trauma plays a central role in behavioral health disorders. Exposure to physically or psychologically harmful or life-threatening events is a common risk factor for both mental and substance use disorders (SAMHSA, 2004). Studies have also linked the experience of trauma to other chronic physical diseases, such as obesity, diabetes and pulmonary diseases (Felitti et al., 1998). Individuals with significant trauma histories are present not only in the behavioral health specialty sector, but in child welfare, criminal and juvenile justice, domestic violence, education and primary and specialty health care. Emerging studies have begun to document positive outcomes in these sectors when trauma is addressed and appropriately treated. SAMHSA has recognized the public health urgency to more systematically address trauma. Investments have been made in the development of education and public awareness materials, screening and assessments, treatment and recovery interventions, and organizational approaches to trauma. Critical to this effort is the development of a workforce trained in trauma-specific or trauma- informed approaches.

In addition, the shift to a recovery-oriented paradigm has resulted in an increased use of peers, recovery support workers, care managers, patient navigators, and health educators. The role of peer specialists is to provide ongoing recovery support for people with mental or substance use disorders. As of September 2011, 23 states have developed certification programs for peer specialists. Certified Peer Specialists/Recovery Coaches may work in many settings including independent recovery community organizations, partial hospitalization or day programs, inpatient or crisis centers, vocational rehabilitation or drop-in centers, residential programs, and medication assisted programs. Peer support activities include self-determination and personal responsibility, providing hope, recovery coaching, life skills, training, communication with providers, health and wellness, illness management, addressing discrimination and promoting full inclusion in the community, assistance with housing, education/employment, and positive social activities (Center for Substance Abuse Treatment [CSAT], 2009; Daniels et al., 2011).

DEMOGRAPHIC INFORMATION

This section will provide data on gender, race and educational level of the mental health and addictions workforce.

Gender

The gender breakdown for some of the major professions working in the field is listed in Table 1.

A sample of 260 Certified Peer Specialists from 28 states found that 33 percent were male and 66 percent were female, and one percent reported they were transgender (Salzer et al., 2010).

Table 1.

Occupation	Male	Female
Psychologists	33.5%	66.5%
Psychiatrists	70%	30%
Social Workers	19.2%	80.8%
Counselors	28.8%	71.2%

Bureau of Labor Statistics, Department of Labor, Occupational Outlook Handbook 2010-11 http://bls.gov/oco/

Similar data were found in several studies that looked at turnover and other staffing issues in the addictions field. These studies reported the percentage of women in the addiction treatment field at 60 percent or higher (Knight et al., 2012; Knudsen et al., 2006; Curtis & Eby, 2010). Information obtained by the International Certification and Reciprocity Consortium (IC&RC) from 15 certification boards[2] reporting on 30,742 counselors found that 61.9 percent were women and 38.1 percent were men (2011).

Racial Composition

Racial and ethnic minorities as a whole comprise approximately 30 percent of the U.S. population (U.S. Census, 2010), and a similar percentage of those receiving services (SAMHSA, 2012; 2008). However, African Americans are represented at a higher rate among service recipients for both mental health and addictions services. As indicated in *Mental Health, United States, 2010* (SAMHSA, 2012a) report, racial minorities account for only:

- 19.2 percent of all psychiatrists;
- 5.1 percent of psychologists;
- 17.5 percent of social workers;
- 10.3 percent of counselors; and
- 7.8 percent of marriage and family therapists.

Information reported from eight certification boards which are members of IC&RC, representing 21,681 counselors as of March 1, 2012, found the racial makeup as described in Table 2 below.

Table 2. Racial Composition

Race	Percent
White	55.8%
Black/African-American	27.9%
Hispanic/Latino	11.1%
American Indian/Alaska Native	0.7%
Asian/Pacific Islander	2.8%

N = 21,681 from 8 boards.

A sample of certified peer specialists found that 21 percent of those respondents were from minority populations (Salzer et al., 2010). The ongoing disparity in the demographics of the workforce and patient population suggest that training in cultural competence will be important.

Education Levels

Dilonardo (2011) reported that almost all states (98 percent) required a master's degree to qualify as a mental health counselor but 45 percent of states did not require any college degree to qualify as a substance abuse counselor. For behavioral health care disciplines, independent practice requires a master's degree in most states; however, for addiction counselors, data available a decade ago indicated that about 50-55 percent of those certified or practicing in the field had at least a master's degree, 75 percent hold a bachelor's degree, and the reminder had either some college, a high school diploma or equivalent (Kaplan, 2003).

WORKFORCE CONDITIONS

This section briefly summarizes some of the major factors that impact the workforce, including high turnover, worker shortages, an aging workforce, inadequate compensation, and recruitment, retention and distribution of the workforce, as well as misperception and prejudice about mental illness and addiction.

High Turnover

Staff turnover is costly in monetary terms with regard to replacement expenses and also disruptive to the therapeutic relationship. SAMHSA's workforce studies (2007, 2006, 2006a) all found high turnover rates reported in the literature at those times. Recent studies corroborate those earlier findings. The 2012 ATTCs workforce survey reported an average annual turnover of addiction services professionals at 18.5 percent across the country (Ryan et.al., 2012). Eby et al. (2010) conducted a study of 739 clinicians over a two-year time period in 27 geographically dispersed public and private treatment organizations and found annual turnover rates of 33.2 percent for counselors and 23.4 percent for clinical supervisors. A study of adolescent treatment programs (Garner et al., 2012) found turnover rates of 31 percent for clinicians and 19 percent for clinical supervisors. These rates are substantially higher when compared to primary care physicians in managed care organizations who had a median turnover rate of approximately seven (7.1) percent (Plomondon et al., 2007). As reported by Anderson (2012), nurse practitioners and physicians assistants had 12 percent turnover rates.

A meta-analysis found that burn-out, stress and lack of social support are antecedents to worker turnover in the social service sector (MorBarak et al., 2001). Other studies found that better opportunities were key reasons for leaving (Eby et al., 2010; Gulf Coast ATTC, 2005). Reported turnover appeared to be worse in rural agencies (Knudsen et al., 2005). Another study by Knight et al. (2012) demonstrated that high turnover produced increased stress and workforce demand for the remaining staff. One study found that clinical supervision reduced emotional exhaustion and turnover intention in counselors working in treatment agencies (Knudsen et al., 2008).

In a Gulf Coast ATTC survey, directors reported annual staff turnover rate was 42 percent. The leading reason for leaving was a better opportunity in the field, followed by personal reasons (illness, family issues, child care, etc.), and inadequate salary. In 2004, program directors in Tennessee reported turnover rates from 15-22 percent. Reported turnover appeared to be higher in rural agencies (Knudsen et al., 2005).

High turnover most often had a negative impact on implementation of evidence-based practices, although some teams were able to use strategies to improve implementation through turnover. Implementation models must consider turbulent behavioral health workforce conditions (Woltmann et al., 2009). Carise et al., (2005) worked with nine community-based treatment centers in Philadelphia to implement a new assessment tool and had trouble recruiting staff for the study due to staff turnover rates of 32 percent among the agencies involved.

Worker Shortages

Concerns about worker shortages have been indicated for a number of years. As reported in *An Action Plan for Behavioral Health Workforce Development* (SAMHSA, 2007), it is projected that by 2020, 12,624 child and adolescent psychologists will be needed but a supply of only 8,312 is anticipated. *Mental Health, United States, 2008* (SAMHSA, 2010), found more than two-thirds of primary care physicians who tried to obtain outpatient mental health services for their patients reported they were unsuccessful because of shortages in mental health care providers, health plan barriers, and lack of coverage or inadequate coverage.

As of March 30, 2012, HRSA reported that there were 3,669 Mental Health, Health Professional Shortage Areas (HPSAs)[3] containing almost 91 million people. It would take 1,846 psychiatrists and 5,931 other practitioners to fill the needed slots. This shortage of workers is not evenly distributed as 55 percent of U.S. counties, all rural, have no practicing psychiatrists, psychologists, or social workers (SAMHSA, 2007). Another study (Thomas et al., 2009) found that 77 percent of counties had a severe shortage of mental health workers, both prescribers and non-prescribers and 96 percent of counties had some unmet need for mental health prescribers.

The two characteristics most associated with unmet need in counties were low per capita income and rural areas.

Ascertaining the supply of addiction treatment workers has been difficult due to a lack of ongoing data collection. In surveys conducted by various regional ATTCs, program directors have indicated problems recruiting adequately prepared staff, often citing at least one or more unfilled full time equivalent (FTE) positions (RMC, 2003; Knudsen et al., 2005). Reasons for recruiting difficulties include insufficient numbers of applicants who meet minimum qualifications (due to lack of experience, certification, or education), a small applicant pool in specific geographic areas, and a lack of interest in the positions due to salary and limited funding (Ryan et al., 2012; Gulf Coast ATTC, 2007). In addition, the Gulf Coast study found that even if all of the 105 positions were filled, 34 percent of agencies would still be understaffed. Agencies reported a need for 56 additional budgeted positions statewide. A survey of agencies in Tennessee conducted by the Central East ATTC (Knudsen et al., 2005) found that program directors reported an average staff shortage of 1.27 FTEs across programs.

Aging Workforce

According to the BLS the median age of various professionals who work in the mental health and addiction field are shown in Table 3 below.

Table 3.

Occupation	Median Age
Psychologists	50.3
Psychiatrists	55.7 (46% are 65+)
Social Workers	42.5
Counselors	42

Bureau of Labor Statistics, Department of Labor, Occupational Outlook Handbook 2010-11 http://bls.gov/oco/

In 2006, more than 50 percent of male U.S. psychiatrists and 25 percent of female psychiatrists were aged 60 or older (SAMHSA, 2010). Recent studies, using samples of hundreds of counselors across programs in many states, reported consistent findings for counselors working in addiction treatment, with an average age in the mid-40s (Knight et al., 2012; Knudsen et al., 2006). The current addiction treatment workforce is middle-aged and even new workers entering the field do so relatively late in their careers (RMC, 2003; RMC, 2003a; National Association for Alcoholism and Drug Abuse Counselors [NAADAC], 2003). Many counselors come into the field as second careers, entering the profession in their mid-forties (SAMHSA, 2006a). Recruiting students into the field, particularly from under represented populations, can serve as a counterbalance to an aging workforce.

Perceptions about Behavioral Health Conditions and Those with Lived Experience

People with mental and substance use disorders often face misunderstanding and discrimination for having these conditions. Those working in the behavioral health field often face the same misperceptions and judgments about their value as clinicians which results in recruitment difficulties and lower pay than comparable fields (National Council of Community Health Centers [NCCBHC], 2011; SAMHSA, 2007; SAMHSA, 2006).

A 2011 compensation study found that the negative beliefs and misunderstandings associated with people suffering mental illnesses and substance use disorders also impacts those working in the field, even as compared to other segments of health care. At a mental health center, a master's level social worker earns $45,344 and an entry level social worker earns $30,000 while in a general health care agency, a social worker earns $50,470. A registered nurse working in a behavioral health organization makes $52,987 while the national average for nurses is $66,530 (NCCBH, 2011).

Most staff in a Northwest Frontier ATTC survey reported that they had lower professional status than other health professionals (RMC, 2003). A series of focus groups throughout New York State indicated that the prejudice and misunderstanding of alcoholism and drug addiction prevents other professions from recognizing and accepting addictions professionals as peers (New York State Office of Alcoholism and Substance Abuse Services [NYS OASAS], 2002).

As discussed in the workforce survey conducted in Texas (Gulf Coast ATTC, 2007), the perception that addictions counselors have low status may also contribute to professionals leaving the field and difficulty in recruiting replacements. Seventy-five percent of directors thought that addictions counselors have lower status than other helping professionals and only four percent thought that addictions counselors have higher status. Among those who thought status was lower, the primary reason was that addictions counselors have less formal education or training.

A number of workforce studies conducted in the past decade found that addiction counselors had lower status than other professionals (NYS OASAS, 2002; RMC, 2003; Gulf Coast ATTC, 2007). Knudsen et al. (2005) also reported that some clinicians may also have lower status due to their own history of substance use disorders. In a series of focus groups conducted primarily with African-American and Hispanic early and mid-career populations, participants stated that addictions treatment was not valued in the larger society and that, therefore, workers were not well compensated or offered supports to avoid burn-out. The lack of information about the field and the perception that the field is not viewed as a valued profession appear to be recruitment barriers for some individuals (Gaumond et al., 2007).

Inadequate Compensation

Compensation for those working in behavioral health is significantly lower than for other health related or other comparable professions. The National Council for Community Behavioral Healthcare (NCCBH) has a membership of over 1,950 community-based, largely non-profit providers delivering both mental health and substance abuse services for persons with mental illness, addictive disorders or both. A 2011 survey conducted by the

NCCBH found a strong positive relationship between salary and organizational size/revenue. In addition, geographic differences in salaries were noted, especially with those in the Northeast when compared to the rest of the county. Also, psychiatrists working in rural settings had higher salaries compared to psychiatrists working in other locations. The NCCBH study also found differences in executive salaries, with the vast majority of executive salaries at mental health centers below $150,000. The average salary of a Chief Executive Officer (CEO) at a community mental health center was $114,247, compared to $136,168 for a CEO at a FQHC. Both of these were significantly less than the top management official at a non-profit hospital, which was $408,927.

This survey also found that salaries for positions in behavioral health care were much lower than reference professions both in other service areas within the health care industry and outside health care. For example, a licensed professional social worker, requiring a Master's degree and typically 2,000 hours of post-graduate experience, earned less than the manager of a fast food restaurant. The median salary for a direct care worker in a 24-hour residential treatment center was $23,000 compared to $25,589, the median salary for an assistant manager at Burger King (NCCBH, 2011).

Compensation for those working in the addictions field is notoriously low. In fact, earlier studies (Kaplan, 2003) suggested that inadequate compensation contributes to high turnover with counselors engaging in significant churning or movement from one job to another to increase their salaries, often by only $1,000 a year. NAADAC (2006) noted that "[m]any of our Addiction Professionals across the USA can currently qualify for food stamps - this is not acceptable - especially if we want quality, competent and long-term professionals." The disparity in the salary for substance abuse counselors and other professional groups is due in part to the difference in credentialing/licensure standards. The lack of national standards for addiction counselors and the absence of any specific degree requirements across many states impact the overall compensation for this group of workers.

Average wages for behavioral health professionals are shown in Table 4.

For comparative purposes, the NCCBH in its 2011 salary survey looked at average salaries for selected professions that required comparable education and training to the professions listed in Table 4 for those disciplines that required a master's degree or less. The selection provides a comparison of average salaries between standard behavioral health professions and allied health/public service workers. These are shown in Table 5.

Table 4. Average Wages from the Bureau of Labor Statistics

Profession	Bureau of Labor Statistics*	National Council Salary Survey
Psychiatrists	$163,660	$168,163
Psychologists	$84,220	$79,900
Marriage & Family Therapists	$49,020	$42,605
Social Worker (MSW)	$50,470	$45,344
Mental Health Counselors (MA)	$41,710	$41,313
Substance Abuse & Behavioral Disorders Counselors (Certified/BA)	$37,030	$34,331

* Bureau of Labor Statistics, - Occupational Outlook Handbook 2009.

Table 5. Average Wages of Reference Professions

Reference Profession	Average Wage
Physician Assistant	$84,830
Physical Therapist	$76,220
Dental Hygienist	$67,860
Secondary School Teacher	$55,150
Subway /Metro Operator	$52,800
Firefighters	$47,270

BLS found similar low wages in Table 6 below.

Table 6.

Profession	Median Wage
Psychiatrists	$164,220
Psychologists	$63,140
Marriage & Family Therapists	$44,590
Mental Health and Substance Abuse Social Workers	$37,210
Substance Abuse & Behavioral Disorders Counselors	$37,030
Mental Health Counselors	$36,810

Bureau of Labor Statistics, Department of Labor, Occupational Outlook Handbook 2010-11 http://bls.gov/oco/

The middle 50 percent of substance abuse and behavioral disorders counselors earned between $29,410 and $47,290. The lowest 10 percent earned less than $24,240, and the highest 10 percent earned more than $59,460. Median annual wages in the industries employing the largest numbers of substance abuse and behavioral disorder counselors were as follows:

A column in an online employment service cited chemical dependency counseling as one of the five most high stress and low paying jobs in the country.[4] The median annual salary it reported was $38,900 with annual salaries ranging from $25,079-$48,517. As reported in this column, many counselors deal with addicted individuals who are often mandated to treatment, and who do not want any interventions.

"While the work can be compelling, substance-abuse counseling ranks as one of the most difficult social work jobs due to its emotional challenges. Watching clients relapse and sometimes become ill or die can take its toll. The combination of being stressed out *and* broke trumps all other career-related gripes." Unfortunately, as with chemical-dependency counselors or parole officers, many of the workers dealing with high stress and low pay provide essential social services. "We can't have a society with no probation officers, no social workers," says Al Lee, director of quantitative analysis at PayScale.com. We should maybe talk about where we want to spend our money as a society" (Leonardi, 2012).

Compensation for Specialty Behavioral Health Providers

Congress determined long ago that community health providers funded by HRSA to serve those without access to other health care and often without insurance should be compensated at cost. These providers receive grants through HRSA and special and higher rates through Medicaid if they are determined to be FQHCs meeting HRSA-determined criteria for service provision and quality. On the other hand, community mental health and substance abuse providers do not have to meet federally determined criteria for service provision and quality. They must meet state certification or credentialing requirements which vary from no special requirements to extensive requirements. These state credentialed providers serve a disproportionate number of low-income and uninsured individuals and are often reimbursed through Medicaid or through state block grants (administered through SAMHSA) at whatever rate or for whatever budget the particular state offers, regardless of the cost of delivering that care.

Table 7. Wages by Setting

Setting	Median Wage
General medical and surgical hospitals	$44,130
Local government	$41,660
Outpatient care centers	$36,650
Individual and family services	$35,210
Residential mental retardation, mental health and substance facilities	$31,300

Bureau of Labor Statistics, Department of Labor, Occupational Outlook Handbook 2010-11 http://bls.gov/oco/

Likewise, community behavioral health is generally not structured as physician-based practices the way private sector practitioners are structured. Hence, the incentives for development and use of health information technology have not been funded for community behavioral health providers as they have for hospitals or practitioner-based providers. The inconsistency in funding for FQHCs and community-based behavioral health care providers makes recruiting and retaining practitioners particularly difficult for these specialty providers serving some of the nation's most-in-need persons with addictions and/or mental illness.

Data on Recruitment, Retention and Distribution

As cited in the major SAMHSA workforce report of 2007, *An Action Plan for Behavioral Health Workforce Development*, "[e]xamining workforce need nationally is complicated by a host of factors. There is no national census on behavioral health workforce that adequately captures the number of trained or employed individuals." As mentioned previously, this lack of data on the workforce has been a major challenge in documenting workforce demand and supply. There is a paucity of information on recruitment. The extensive SAMHSA 2007 Action Plan report found that the existing literature focused on engaging minorities in graduate-level training. Recruitment efforts are not well documented and little data exists on results of recruitment initiatives. Some workforce studies that were conducted specifically on the addiction workforce reported that staff recruitment was hampered by low salaries as cited by a majority of program directors surveyed (RMC, 2003; RMC, 2003a; NYS OASAS, 2002). Management staff also reported that candidates often did not meet the minimum job requirements due to lack of training and education or experience in substance abuse treatment. In a workforce report conducted in

Texas in 2007, program directors cited the primary reasons for recruiting difficulties are insufficient numbers of applicants who meet minimum qualifications due to lack of experience, certification, or education (Gulf Coast ATTC, 2007).

More literature exists on retention of staff; however, most of the literature focuses only on the addiction services workforce. In these studies, the turnover rates range from 18.5 percent (Knudsen et al., 2003) to over 50 percent (McLellan et al., 2003). Kaplan (2003) found that inadequate compensation contributed to high turnover of addiction counselors which resulted in movement from one job/agency to another in search of salary increases.

Growth across the behavioral health professions is not consistent. As cited in *Mental Health, United States*, 2002 (Sullivan et al., 2004), an increase in the number of both psychologists and social workers has been noted for years, and, as noted on page 12, the number of psychiatrists has been stable and therefore not keeping up with the growth in population. As Table 8 demonstrates, the projected growth identified by the BLS for behavioral health occupations is in many cases greater than the average for most occupations. Given that there are many reports that cite workforce shortages for addiction counselors, it is clear that strategies need to be developed to address the field's recruitment issues.

Table 8. Projected Growth of Specific Occupations

Profession	2008 Workforce	2018 Projection	Increase
Substance Abuse & Behavioral Disorders Counselors*	86,100	104,200	18,100 (21%)
Mental Health Counselors*	113,000	140,400	27,200 (24%)
Mental Health & Substance Abuse Social Workers	137,300	164,100	26,800 (20%)
Psychologists	152,000	168,800	16,800 (11%)
Marriage and Family Therapists	27,300	31,300	3,900 (14%)

* Projected growth rate much higher than average for other professions. Bureau of Labor Statistics, Department of Labor, Occupational Outlook Handbook 2010-11 http://bls.gov/oco/

The CEO of NAADAC addressed the issue of recruitment, retention and reimbursement in a 2006 commentary entitled *Blueprint for the States: Policies to Improve the Way States Organize and Deliver Alcohol and Drug Prevention Treatment* (Tuohy, 2006). In this *Blueprint*, Tuohy calls for increased understanding of addiction as a disease and increased attention to incentive such as loan repayments and forgiveness, specifically for addictions counselors, as key ingredients for success in recruitment. Tuohy also calls for adequate rewards as careers progress, with promotions and recognition, as well as assistance for addictions counselors to remain up-to- date on the latest advances in the addiction treatment and recovery field in order to retain a highly qualified workforce. Finally, Tuohy recognizes the need for adequate compensation and therefore higher rates of reimbursement for addictions professionals. Tuohy discusses the lack of common national standards or competing standards for key professional areas, especially for addictions professionals, while calling on multiple credentialing bodies to work together toward core competencies that could be widely accepted.

As noted in the aforementioned demographic information, the majority of behavioral health workers are white females in their mid-40s. In its publication, *In the Nation's Compelling Interest: Ensuring Diversity in the Health-Care Workforce,* the IOM (2004) reported that racial and ethnic minority health care professionals are significantly more likely than their white peers to serve minority and medically underserved communities, which would improve problems of limited minority access to care. This report also cites studies that found that minority patients who have a choice are more likely to select health care professionals of their own racial or ethnic background, and that they are generally more satisfied with the care that they receive from minority professionals.

There is also a significant mal-distribution of workers. As found by Greiner and Knebel (2003), behavioral health professionals are in short supply in rural and low income communities. In fact, 55 percent of U.S. counties – all rural – do not have any practicing behavioral health workers. And, as reported earlier, more than three-quarters of counties in the United States have a serious shortage of mental health professionals (Thomas,et al.,2009). Data on the distribution of peers working in either rural or urban areas are not available at this time. Though there is some information about peer specialists, the information is limited in scope.

Data are available on a number of variables for the major disciplines comprising the workforce providing services for persons with mental or substance use disorders. However, these data can only be obtained from a variety of sources. No single source of workforce data, either discipline specific or on a national level, exists that details the demographics, supply, demand or practice information.

Special Issues of the Prevention Workforce

Particularly difficult issues confront the prevention workforce in behavioral health. Underpinning some of these issues are different models of what constitutes prevention. In the 1950s, public health classified preventive measures in three basic categories, primary, secondary, and tertiary. But in the 1980s, Dr. Robert Gordon proposed a new Operational Classification of Disease Prevention (1983), which restricted "the use of the term 'preventive' to measures, actions, or interventions that are practiced by or on persons who are not, at the time, suffering from any discomfort or disability due to the disease or condition being prevented." As articulated by Gordon and reiterated by the Institute of Medicine in 2004 in the context of behavioral health, these approaches may be for the whole population (universal prevention), for selected sub-populations (selective prevention) or at-risk individuals (indicated) prevention. The implementation of this model in behavioral health depends on a data-driven continuum of evidence-based services.

The lack of a wide-spread understanding of the primary prevention model and the role of prevention in behavioral health leads to a concomitant lack of priority given to funding prevention activities which are evidence-based, well-documented, and known to be both efficacious and cost-effective. The effect of this disparity is cumulative: low salaries force many qualified individuals to leave the field; high staff turnover creates the need for additional training; the cost of training can be prohibitive for programs and individuals.

An additional challenge for prevention professionals is the lack of a national standard for credentialing. Despite the existence of the International Certification Reciprocity Consortium/Alcohol and Other Drug Abuse which provides certification of competency for prevention specialists, state and local programs may use their own certification standards or impose no standards at all. This lack of standardization is compounded by the fact that states vary significantly in their prevention approaches – some are bringing behavioral health and primary care under one roof while others have substance abuse prevention programs within public health or mental illness prevention integrated into specialty mental health services – which further complicates the question of creating one national certification standard to apply across the board.

Impact of Affordable Care Act and MHPAEA on the Behavioral Health Workforce

In 2014, up to 38 million more Americans will have an opportunity to be covered by health insurance due to changes under the Affordable Care Act (Congressional Budget Office [CBO], 2010; SAMHSA, 2011). Between 20 to 30 percent of these people (as many as 11 million) may have a serious mental illness or serious psychological distress, and/or a substance use disorder (SAMHSA, 2011). Among the currently uninsured aged 22 to 64 with family income of less than 150 percent of the federal poverty level, 36.8 percent had illicit drug or alcohol dependence/abuse or mental illness (SAMHSA, 2011). However, the Supreme Court decision on June 28, 2012 gave the states the option to expand Medicaid as stipulated in the Affordable Care Act. The CBO therefore reduced by 6 million the number of people who may be covered by Medicaid and the Children's Health Insurance Program (CBO, 2012).

This growth in the number of people who will be identified with a mental or substance use disorder requires an expanded workforce. However, the composition of the workforce will be reshaped by the Affordable Care Act with the move toward more integrated primary and behavioral health care. New integrated care structures such as accountable care organizations and health homes funded or promoted by the Affordable Care Act offer new opportunities for persons with behavioral health conditions, and will necessitate additional training for primary care workers as well as new specialty practitioners as part of the multi-disciplinary teams. Brief interventions and brief treatment will likely be delivered by staff in primary care settings as screening for depression, alcohol and substance abuse becomes a standard part of care. Staff will include health educators, nurse practitioners, care managers, physicians as well as counselors, social workers, psychologists, and addiction specialists.

Primary care settings differ from the specialty sector. As integration of primary and behavioral health services becomes the standard, there will be a greater emphasis on evidence-based practices and outcomes, especially in light of the HHS National Quality Strategy and SAMHSA's National Behavioral Health Quality Framework which are focused on improving quality of care as well as improving both administrative and clinical processes.

People with more severe and persistent mental and substance use disorders will receive longer term and more intensive treatment, either within a primary care setting or specialty setting. The use of peers to promote long-term recovery is also expanding across the country. These peer specialists, who in some states are now being certified, play a key role in the recovery process serving as role models, navigators, recovery coaches, as well as providing hope, a critical part of the recovery process. These peer specialists are also an important addition to the workforce to help meet the need for services and supports that can be provided by trained persons who are certified but not licensed as traditional health or behavioral health care practitioners.

Creative retooling and repurposing of the existing behavioral health workforce will be required to support integration, with some workers in significantly expanded and changed roles with broader competencies. Great strides will need to be made in the adoption of evidence-based practices, team work skills and collaboration. In primary care setting a team–based approach is used which requires more flexibility in scheduling. New or expanded roles and types of workers are also likely to be needed to facilitate integration, including health educators, behavioral health specialists, and care managers (SAMHSA, 2011).

ENUMERATION OF NEEDS

A number of challenges await the workforce over the next several years. As discussed above, both the demand for services and where services are delivered will change in the coming years. The rise in the use of medications for mental and substance use disorders as well as the integration of care are reshaping who and how services are provided. The use of psychotropic medications has grown exponentially over the past decade. Mojtabai and Olfson (2011) found that antidepressants are the third most prescribed class of medications in the country. However, often these patients are not clearly diagnosed or referred for further assessment as primary care physicians are concerned about a diagnosis that could result in prejudice for the patient and lack of easy access to mental health and addiction professionals. The use of medication assisted addiction treatment is also increasing (SAMHSA, 2011).

Integrated care is predicated on a holistic, public health care model requiring a team approach to primary and behavioral health services. Integrated care will bring additional challenges to the field. Requirements for licensure/certification are not standardized across states and include little, if any, preparation related to physical health conditions or working in primary care settings. National core competencies for behavioral health care are lacking. Practice will be based on science; employing evidence-based approaches will become the norm. However, the adoption of evidenced-based practices still often has a lag time of about 15-20 years. The majority of members of the core primary disciplines (physicians, nurses, social workers, psychologists, physicians' assistants and others) are also likely to have insufficient training in behavioral health.

In addition, the need for and adoption of interoperable electronic health records and other health information technology is changing practice and increasing the accountability for quality. All of these issues indicate successful integration of care will be predicated on comprehensive training for all staff involved in providing services, whether in primary or specialty care settings and whether in traditional or multi-disciplinary practices.

The prevalence of co-occurring mental and substance use disorders has been documented in the 2010 NSDUH. The findings indicate that 45.1 percent (9.2 million) of the 20.3 million adults with substance use disorders also had a mental illness as compared to 17.6 percent without a substance use disorder. Of the 45.9 million adults who had any mental illness, 20 percent or 9.2 million had a co-occurring substance use disorder. Comparatively, 11.2 million or 6.1 percent of adults with a substance use disorder did not have a mental illness in the past year (SAMHSA, 2011). This underscores the need for the development and promotion of behavioral health competencies among both the addictions and the mental health workforce.

As the use of medication assisted treatment increases and treatment for co-occurring disorders becomes more frequent, employment of physicians in behavioral health settings may increase. Physicians in primary care are also more likely to be prescribing such medications and treating individuals with addictions. The use of physicians also increases the likelihood that primary care will be delivered onsite in community mental health and substance abuse facilities. In a recent study, almost 75 percent of the participating substance abuse treatment organizations indicated that finding a physician in the local community who had experience treating substance use disorders was somewhat or very difficult. More importantly, inadequate funding for physicians' services was negatively associated with the employment of physicians (Knudsen et al., 2012). Physicians report barriers to the use of medication assisted treatment and screening and brief intervention, including not feeling comfortable in managing all components of either type of intervention (Dilonardo, 2011).

Meeting the country's behavioral health needs requires a sufficient supply of well trained, competent workforce. Given the issues discussed in this paper there are some strategies that will help us achieve the promise of better outcomes for people with and at risk for mental and substance use disorders. These may include:

- Promoting cross training for the behavioral health workforce to enhance capabilities to serve individuals with co-occurring disorders and how to work in complex multi- disciplinary teams;
- Fostering the expansion of the workforce by recruiting a more diverse workforce and concentrating on underserved populations. Specific populations that need additional services include children and adolescents, geriatric patients, and those living in rural areas. Increasing the use of consumers/persons in recovery, parent/family, and other peers, as well as paraprofessionals and practitioner extenders;
- Disseminating and promoting the adoption of evidence-based practices to reduce the delay in adoption of science-based interventions including ongoing supervision to ensure treatment fidelity;
- Encouraging the development and dissemination of behavioral health core competencies for the primary and other health care workforce;
- Providing training and education on recovery-oriented care and recovery principles for the behavioral health field; and
- Developing standardized workforce data collection elements that can be collected and analyzed on a regular basis to assist in gathering demographic, setting and practice information.

SAMHSA AND HRSA WORKFORCE INITIATIVES

SAMHSA and HRSA each fund workforce initiatives that address many of the challenges facing the behavioral health field. These initiatives provide a broad range of activities that address the needs of the current workforce and provide support for future growth.

On June 5, 2012, SAMHSA and HRSA Administrators held a joint listening session with key behavioral health field leaders. From that session, a consensus emerged about many issues that need to be tackled if the behavioral health workforce is to keep pace with the growing need and rapidly changing health care environment.

This portion of the report is divided into two sections. The first highlights SAMHSA's and HRSA's current workforce programs and other activities to advance the behavioral health workforce, and the second describes workforce collaborations between SAMHSA and HRSA, including results from the joint listening session. Note that for programs spending only a portion of their funds on workforce development activities. The FY 2012 funding levels provided are approximate. Expenditures of FY 2012 funds may vary during project execution in order to be responsive to emerging program needs (e.g., in a given year, a cohort of grantees may or may not demonstrate a need for technical assistance on workforce development).

SAMHSA Workforce Programs

Addiction Technology Transfer Centers

The ATTC network, which was first funded in 1993, consisted of 14 regional centers and one national coordinating center in the cohort that ended in FY 2011. They provide services in all 50 states, the District of Columbia, Puerto Rico and the Caribbean Basin, and the Pacific Islands. The purpose of this program is to develop and strengthen the workforce that provides addiction treatment services. The ATTCs partner with substance abuse Single State Authorities, treatment provider associations, addiction counselors, multidisciplinary professionals, faith and recovery community leaders, family members of those in recovery, and other stakeholders to: (1) raise awareness of evidence-based and promising treatment and recovery practices; (2) build skills to prepare the workforce to deliver state-of-the-art addiction treatment and recovery services; (3) and change practice by incorporating these new skills into everyday use for the purpose of improving addiction treatment and recovery outcomes. For the first time in its history, the ATTC network has conducted a national workforce survey to obtain information on the state of the current workforce.

This survey, *Vital Signs: Taking the Pulse of the Addiction Treatment Profession* (Ryan, Murphy, & Krom, 2012), provides an overview of the characteristics and workforce development needs of the substance use disorders treatment field.

The data collection process included a survey of clinical directors; telephone interviews with a selected group of clinical directors; telephone interviews with thought leaders; and a review of existing literature and data sets. The 57-item instrument survey was distributed by ATTC Regional Centers to a sample of 631 programs drawn from the Inventory of Substance Abuse Treatment Services using a dual sampling method to ensure that data would be both nationally and regionally representative. The response rate was 88 percent.

A summary of the national findings about the substance abuse workforce as identified by the ATTC survey is described below.

Basic Demographics of the Substance Abuse workforce
- Sixty-five percent of clinical directors had at least a master's degree and they have, on average, 17 years of experience in the field. Seventy-seven percent are state licensed or certified. About one third are identified as being in recovery from a substance use disorder.
- Thirty-six percent of direct care staff had a Master's degree, and 24 percent had a bachelor's degree as their highest level of education. The majority of direct care staff is currently licensed/certified or seeking licensure/certification. Slightly less than one-third of direct care staff are in recovery from substance use disorders as estimated by their clinical directors.
- Almost one-third of clinical directors are only somewhat proficient in web-based technologies, and almost half of substance use disorder facilities do not have an electronic health record system in place.

Common Strategies and Methodologies to Prepare, Retain, and Maintain the Substance Abuse workforce
- Substance use disorder treatment facilities most commonly offer professional development for staff through new employee orientation, ongoing training, and direct supervision. When facilities do not provide for staff training and continuing education, the most commonly reported reason was a lack of funds.
- The majority of survey respondents reported that staff at their facility had been trained in both culturally responsive and gender responsive substance use disorder treatment.
- Clinical directors interviewed emphasized the positive effects that developing relationships with colleges and universities can have on recruiting qualified professionals.

In order to achieve the major goals, the ATTCs utilize technology transfer as a systematic process through which skills, techniques, models and approaches emanating from research are translated, disseminated and adopted by practitioners. They also develop curricula standards for pre-service and academic programs which are compatible with and support SAMHSA's Addiction Counseling Competencies (CSAT, 2006; 2007) and provide a coordinated approach to the training and technology transfer needs of clinical supervisors. ATTCs develop and disseminate educational materials and resources on substance use treatment. They also collaborate on developing and supporting emerging leaders in the field.

Another critical component of technology transfer is to reduce the time it takes for evidence- based practices to be adopted by practitioners. Toward that end, SAMHSA and the National Institute on Drug Abuse (NIDA) have an inter-agency agreement (IAA) to facilitate cooperative effort that foster the timely transfer and implementation of research-based findings from NIDA-conducted research, including NIDA's Clinical Trials Network. Through this IAA, NIDA transfers $1.5 million each year to SAMHSA for the ATTCs to support the NIDA/SAMHSA Blending Initiative. Begun in 2001, this project is designed to meld science and practice together to improve substance use disorder treatment and accelerate the dissemination of research-based drug abuse treatment findings into community-based practice.

There are three components to the Blending Initiative:

- *Blending Conferences* – Each is designed to enhance bidirectional communication between researchers, clinical practitioners, and policy-makers regarding innovative scientific findings about drug abuse and addiction.
- *State Agency Partnerships* – NIDA works closely with federal and state policy-makers to help identify strategies to accelerate the adoption of science-based practices.
- *Development of Products and Tools* – Blending Teams composed of members from the ATTC Network, NIDA researchers, and community treatment providers participating in NIDA's Clinical Trials Network, are convened to design user-friendly tools or "products" that are based on recently tested NIDA research.

These products are introduced to treatment providers to facilitate the adoption of science-based interventions in their communities at nearly the same time that research results are published in peer-reviewed journals.

The ATTC Network touches many people working in the addiction services field, which is attested to by the following data taken from 2010:

- ATTC Network listserv has over 57,000 subscribers.
- There were 987 events with 26,655 participants.
- One hundred eighty-five products accessible on the ATTC Network Websites received 19,940 downloads.
- The ATTC Web site had almost a million (979,680) unique visits and many people visited more than once as there were 2,612,592 total views.

The ATTC program was re-competed in 2012 with 10 geographic ATTCs reflecting the 10 HHS geographic regions, four specialty ATTCS for (1) SBIRT; (2) HIT in Rural Areas; (3) American Indians and Alaska Natives; and (4) Hispanic and Latino Issues and a National Coordinating Center. Funding for the ATTC program was $9,081,000 in FY 2011 and $9,064,000 in FY 2012.

Partners for Recovery

Partners for Recovery (PFR) is an initiative sponsored by SAMHSA to address issues of national significance with respect to recovery, cross-systems collaboration, workforce development, leadership development, and promotion of accurate perceptions of addiction and mental illness and those who experience these conditions. The PFR Initiative supports and provides technical resources to those who deliver services related to the prevention and treatment of substance use disorders and co-occurring mental health disorders and seeks to build capacity and improve services and systems of care. One of PFR's core activities is developing and implementing a comprehensive strategy to address workforce issues for the addiction treatment and recovery field. Below are the workforce activities that PFR supported in FY 2011.

- *Advanced Leadership Institute* – The Advanced Leadership Institute (ALI) was designed to enhance the leadership development skills of emerging leaders in the addiction field. An objective of the program is to further the development of leaders to impact policy and systems change. This 11-month program trained 28 leaders from across the nation. Leaders' skills are enhanced through an extensive set of development experiences, including individual assessments, an intensive four-day Leader Development Immersion Session, ongoing

coaching, a mid-year two-day Booster (i.e., follow-up) Session, and a sophisticated knowledge- and skill-application project. This programming is all supported by a suite of online and print resources available via a site tailored to meet the particular needs of ALI leaders and their coaches. *FY 2011 Budget $510,000.*
- *School for Prevention Leadership* – The School for Prevention Leadership was specifically designed to bolster the substance abuse prevention workforce and to contribute to the professionalization of the field. The School includes a class of 24 scholars, who were competitively selected from across the country. This 10-month program consists of individual and team assessments, a week-long immersion training, a two-and-a-half day re-immersion training, mentoring, and a graduation. *FY 2011 Budget $336,000.*
- *Environmental Scan on Certification for Peer Specialists and Recovery Coaches* – PFR conducted a study to create a more complete picture of the number of, and process for developing, recovery coaches and certified peer specialists, and to facilitate states' readiness for the Affordable Care Act implementation. The report provides information about states that currently have a certification and training process for peer support service provision, the states' expectations concerning competencies, use of a defined curriculum, and the funding streams for these services. The report also provides information concerning Medicaid billing for peer service delivery and the barriers that impede Medicaid reimbursement. Because the Affordable Care Act will result in an increased demand for services for substance use disorders, the use of peer specialists/recovery coaches can help meet the demand for increased services and promote recovery management. *FY 2011 Budget $56,900.*
- *Lonnie E. Mitchell Historically Black Colleges and Universities Behavioral Health Policy Academy* – The 4th Annual Dr. Lonnie E. Mitchell Historically Black Colleges and Universities (HBCU) Behavioral Health Policy Academy provided a unique forum to promote behavioral health on HBCU campuses and build workforce capacity to address the behavioral health needs of the American public. This policy academy offered a framework for facilitated team discussions to support proposed mini-grant implementation plans. Teams left the Policy Academy with action plans for implementing their mini-grant projects and creating sustainable systems of change on their campuses. The Academy continues the legacy and work of

the late Dr. Lonnie E. Mitchell, an accomplished educator, administrator, policy advisor and psychotherapist. The 21 mini-grant recipients who attended this conference were charged with the following activities during the conference: (1) review campus-specific projects related to identified behavioral health priorities; (2) refine proposed activities to ensure sustainable outcomes; and (3) identify opportunities for collaboration and confirm implementation strategies. *FY 2011 Budget $390,000.*

The total budget for the workforce initiatives under PFR was $1,292,900 in FY 2011. SAMHSA estimates based on planned activities that the total budget for the workforce initiatives under PFR is $300,000 for FY 2012. The funding is from two budget lines: (1) CSAT Program of Regional and National Significance (PRNS) Program Coordination and Evaluation; and, (2) CSAT PRNS Special Initiatives/Outreach.

Historically Black Colleges and Universities – Center for Excellence in Behavioral Health at Morehouse School of Medicine

The HBCU- Center for Excellence (HBCU-CFE) has three major goals which encompass promoting behavioral health to positively impact student retention, expanding campus service capacity, including the provision of culturally appropriate behavioral health resources, and facilitating best practices dissemination and behavioral health workforce development. Though the latter goal most directly relates to workforce development, the workforce development tasks assigned to the HBCU-CFE are:

- Promoting evidence-based and emerging best practices in behavioral health and disseminating information about effective practices to member institutions;
- Facilitating on-site and distance learning opportunities for HBCU students and faculty in behavioral health and workforce development, leadership, and other related activities;
- Facilitating the mentoring of students by schools and highlighting model programs in behavioral health;
- Partnering with programs for regional and local training initiatives with tracks specifically addressing HBCUs; and
- Promoting awareness and access to behavioral health resources, SAMHSA's publications and web-based material and other related resources.

In addition, a number of specific activities performed by the HBCU-CFE that are directed toward enhancing the capability and capacity of the workforce include the following:

- Enhance workforce development opportunities through partnerships with community- based providers and organizations.
- Increase the number of HBCU students interning in the behavioral health field.
- Increase HBCU student exposure to career options in the behavioral health workforce.
- Establish and/or increase HBCU partnerships with local, regional and state entities committed to increasing diversity in the behavioral health workforce.

Funding for the HBCU-CFE in FY 2011 was $1.5 million. Funding for the HBCU-CFE in FY 2012 was $500,000.

Minority Fellowship Program

The objective of the Minority Fellowship Programs (MFP) is to increase the knowledge of issues related to mental health conditions and addictions among minorities, and to improve the quality of mental health services and substance abuse prevention and treatment delivered to ethnic minority populations. SAMHSA provides grants to encourage and facilitate the doctoral and post-doctoral development of nurses, psychiatrists, social workers, psychologists, marriage and family therapists, and professional counselors by providing funding to organizations which oversee the fellowship opportunities.

Program goals are to support doctoral training in mental health and substance abuse services by:

- Promoting culturally competent mental health and substance abuse services provided to ethnic minority populations;
- Increasing the number of professionals delivering mental health and substance abuse services to ethnic minority populations; and
- Increasing the general knowledge and research of issues related to ethnic minority and substance abuse treatment.

The MFP increases the pool of professionals qualified to provide leadership, consultation, training, and administration to government and public and private organizations concerned with the development and implementation of programs and services for under-served ethnic minority persons with mental and/or substance use disorders. In FY 2011, there were 120 fellows in the MFP and, of those, six reported they are planning to specialize in the substance use disorders field.

In 2011, SAMHSA funded a three-year program which awarded five grants for a total amount of $4,073,000, from the Center for Mental Health Services (CMHS; $3,455,000), Center for Substance Abuse Prevention (CSAP; $71,000), and CSAT ($547,000). In 2012, SAMHSA awarded five continuation grants and one new grant to include professional counselors in the program for a total amount of $4,975,941, from CMHS ($4,388,665), CSAP ($67,471), and CSAT ($519,807).

Knowledge Application Program

SAMHSA's Knowledge Application Program (KAP) addresses the knowledge application needs of behavioral health treatment providers by synthesizing, publishing, and disseminating substance abuse treatment and related mental health best practices.

KAP serves as a primary source of information dissemination on strategies, best practices, and protocols for service delivery by the workforce. KAP is responsible for identifying target audiences for the SAMHSA products, tailoring products to the specific needs of those audiences, and developing specialized marketing plans for the products to ensure the appropriate information is transmitted to the right audience in the most effective format in a timely manner. It is supported by follow-on activities which help the intended audience use the information.

Among the products developed by KAP are the Treatment Improvement Protocols (TIPs) and the TIP collateral products; Technical Assistance Publications (TAPs), independent publications on topics such as *Anger Management*, *Substance Abuse Relapse Prevention for Older Adults*, and *Brief Counseling for Marijuana Dependence*; and many consumer publications/brochures. In 2011, the KAP program:

- Cleared and printed two TIPS;
- Produced 41 TIP collateral and other materials including Quick Guides, KAP Keys, and Consumer booklets;
- Produced and disseminated five Advisories and a *SAMHSA In Brief*;
- Produced a DVD with three family education videos;
- Continued the development of eight TIPS and two TAPs; and
- Started the development of one new TIP.

In addition, KAP is moving ahead with strategies in knowledge dissemination using modern technology.

SAMHSA funding for the KAP program was $3,893,339 in FY 2011. SAMHSA funding for the KAP program was $2,500,000 in FY 2012. The funding for the KAP for FY 2012 is from: CSAT PRNS Screening for Brief Intervention and Referral Treatment, Targeted Capacity Expansion-General, Post Partum Women, Access to Recovery, Children & Families, Treatment Systems for Homelessness, Minority AIDs Initiative, Opioid Treatment Programs/Regulatory Activities, Substance Abuse Prevention and Treatment and Block Grant-Set Aside.

Screening, Brief Intervention and Referral to Treatment Medical Residency Program

General medicine physicians are positioned to play a critical role in the recognition and treatment of patients with, or at risk for, substance use disorders. Since its inception in 2008, the SBIRT Medical Residency Program's primary purpose has been to develop and implement training programs to teach medical residents skills to provide evidence-based screening, brief intervention, brief treatment and referral to specialty treatment for patients who have, or are at risk for, a substance use disorder. Another purpose of the program is to promote adoption of SBIRT through delivery of training to local and statewide medical communities for wider dissemination of SBIRT practices. This program promotes systemic change in residency programs by integrating SBIRT into the curriculum on a long-term basis so that SBIRT will be a component of the education provided to each successive class of medical residents. SBIRT Medical Residency Program grant funds are used to develop SBIRT curricula and clinical training as part of residency programs for physicians in primary care to include family medicine, internal medicine, obstetrics and gynecology, pediatrics, emergency medicine, trauma, psychiatry and others. In 2011, there were 17 medical residency programs participating in the program.

In 2011, 1,335 residents were trained through the Medical Residency grant program, with a total of 3,998 trained to date. In addition, grantees have trained 1,944 non-residents (e.g., physician assistants, psychologists, social workers, other health care professionals) during the 2011 reporting period, and 8,572 since 2008.

In 2011, the SBIRT Medical Residency program was funded at $5,865,000. In 2012, the SBIRT Medical Residency program was funded at $6,221,000.

Prescribing Opioids for Chronic Pain

SAMHSA'S courses on "Prescribing Opioids for Chronic Pain: Balancing Safety & Efficacy" are designed for primary care physicians, as well as dentists and oral surgeons, advance practice nurses, and physician assistants. They were developed in consultation with the American Academy of Pain Medicine and an independent panel of experts in medical education, pharmacology, pain management, regulation, and addiction. The courses are approved for 6.5 hours of Category one credit under the Physician Recognition AwardTM program of the American Medical Association, as well the accreditation programs of the American Academy of Family Physicians and the American Osteopathic Association. Topics addressed in this training include evidence-based strategies for patient selection, risk assessment, and patient education, factors in selecting an appropriate opioid, techniques for effective patient monitoring, and knowledge of why and how to stop prescribing opioids and management of the patient with a different approach.

Courses are delivered in face-to-face training sessions and are also available online. Through September 2011, courses have been delivered at 40 sites in the continental U.S. and Alaska and have reached more than 6,000 health professionals. Special versions of the course have been developed for military medical personnel and staff of the Indian Health Service. Actual attendance at the 12 courses delivered between October 1, 2010, and September 29, 2011, was 1,478. In addition, an estimated 1,800 physicians have viewed recordings of the live courses that are posted on the sponsors' websites or distributed on DVDs. During this same time period, more than 2,500 registrants had completed at least one online course, and over 3,000 separate course certificates had been issued.

For FY 2011, the cost to conduct seven live and three online courses was $350,000. For FY 2012, the cost is $350,000.

Physician Clinical Support System for the Treatment of Substance Use Disorders

The Physician Clinical Support System (PCSS) is a national project to support physicians who are treating opioid dependent persons with methadone or buprenorphine. In July 2011, SAMHSA awarded the PCSS for Opioid Therapies, to the American Academy of Addiction Psychiatry. The purpose of this grant is to develop a free national mentoring network that will provide clinical support (e.g., clinical updates, consultations, evidence-based outcomes, and training) to physicians, dentists and other medical professionals in the appropriate use of opioids for the treatment of chronic pain and opioid-related addiction. This initiative contributes to SAMHSA's efforts to address the nationwide issue of morbidity and mortality caused by misuse/abuse and fatal drug interactions involving opioids used in the treatment of addiction and chronic pain. The target population for the clinical support system includes primary care physicians, pain specialists, psychiatrists, and other non-addiction medical practitioners who treat opioid dependent patients and are less familiar with opioid dependence treatment than addiction specialists. In addition, addiction specialists will also be encouraged to participate in the PCSS or serve as mentors for physicians desiring to treat opioid dependent patients with buprenorphine products.

In FY 2011, funding for this program was $500,000. In FY 2012, funding for this program was $500,000.

Physician Clinical Support System-Opioids

The purpose of the PCSS-Opioids grant is to develop a free national mentoring network that will provide clinical support (e.g., clinical updates, consultations, evidence-based outcomes and training) to physicians, dentists, and other medical professionals in the appropriate use of opioids for the treatment of chronic pain and opioid-related addiction. This initiative is targeted to prescribers (physicians, dentists) and other health professionals working in SAMHSA-certified opioid treatment programs as well as those prescribers using opiate-based therapy for chronic pain. The training and clinical support provided under this initiative address the specific complexities that are inherent in opioid-based therapy and the ways in which those complexities affect the appropriate care of individuals being treated for chronic pain and opioid-related addiction.

The PCSS-Opioids grant funds are used primarily to support infrastructure development, including the following types of activities:

- Establish and maintain a cadre of expert clinicians and educators to provide support for qualified health care providers preparing for, or engaging in, opioid use in treatment of chronic pain and opioid-related addiction;
- Disseminate authoritative and standardized clinical materials and clinical tools;
- Promote PCSS-Opioids services to identified target populations;
- Provide mentoring support, observation of practice, and consultative services by phone and e-mail that promote and support qualified

health care providers in the use of opioids in the treatment of opioid-related addiction and chronic pain; and
- Educate prospective practitioners through web site (educational webinars) and published resources, such as TIPS containing science-based best practice guidelines for the treatment and maintenance of patients with opioid dependency and chronic pain.

Funding was provided to the following groups: American Academy of Addiction Psychiatry; American Osteopathic Academy of Addiction Medicine; American Psychiatric Association, American Dental Association, American Society for Pain Management Nursing, and International Nurses Society on Addictions.

In FY 2011, funding for this program was $500,000. In FY 2012, funding for this program was $500,000. In FY 2011, this program was funded from the Opioid Treatment Programs/Regulatory Activities budget. In FY 2012, this program was funded from the Opioid Treatment Programs/Regulatory Activities budget.

Prevention Fellowship Program

The Prevention Fellowship Program, funded by the SAMHSA's CSAP, was launched in 2006 as an effort to build a workforce of substance abuse prevention professionals. The Prevention Fellowship Program addresses workforce development issues in the substance abuse prevention field by:

- Addressing the challenges facing the substance abuse field, including barriers to effective staff recruitment and retention, low wages, high turnover, inconsistent training and credentialing, and aging worker retirements;
- Providing opportunities for individuals to strengthen and apply knowledge gained through their academic programs and work experience in prevention service programs, sharpen their skills, and develop strong networks among a range of other public health professionals; and
- Covering all of the cross-cutting principles in the SAMHSA Strategic Plan through formal educational experiences, training, work experience, coaching, mentoring, and research/literature review.

The 103 fellows, who have participated in the Prevention Fellowship Program since its inception in 2006, represent 43 states, six U.S. territories, and two national organizations that support substance abuse prevention systems. Of the four completed cohorts from 2006 through 2009, 74 participants have enrolled in the program and over 70 percent have graduated. Of the program graduates, 85 percent have become certified by the IC&RC. Post fellowship employment data indicate that over 45 percent of fellows have pursued positions and/or post graduate education in the prevention field. There were 15 fellows in the FY 2011 cohort.

FY 2011 funding was $1,691,284 for the Prevention Fellows Program. FY 2012 funding was $1,058,771 for the Prevention Fellows Program. This program is funded from the CSAP PRNS Strategic Prevention Framework.

Recovery to Practice Initiative

This initiative seeks to advance a recovery-oriented approach to mental health care by developing, promoting, and disseminating training curricula on how to translate the concept of mental health recovery into practice; and by providing a Recovery to Practice (RTP) Recovery Resource Center for mental health professionals engaged in this work. The RTP initiative includes two complementary components: (1) creating a Recovery Resource Center for mental health professionals complete with web-based and print materials, training, and technical assistance for professionals engaged in the transformation process; and (2) creating and disseminating recovery-oriented training materials for each of the major mental health professions. Through these two major components, the RTP initiative aims to foster a better understanding of recovery, recovery-oriented practices, and the roles of the various professions in promoting recovery.

The national mental health professional organizations that are receiving funding to develop recovery-oriented educational materials and train thousands of psychiatrists, psychologists, psychiatric nurses, social workers, and mental health peer specialists are: American Psychiatric Association, American Psychological Association, American Psychiatric Nurses Association, Council on Social Work Education, and National Association of Peer Specialists. In addition to these organizations, beginning in 2011, NAADAC has also been included as a key partner in the Recovery to Practice initiative.

With recovery-oriented training materials, mental health professionals will be able to embrace and practice recovery-oriented approaches while enhancing their core personal and professional values. In addition, they will learn new ways of working collaboratively across professions to more effectively support individuals with mental illnesses in entering into and pursuing recovery.

In FY 2011, the funding was $836,000. In FY 2012, the funding was $1,030,000.

Mental Health Care Provider Education in HIV/AIDS Program

The Mental Health Care Provider Education (MHCPE) in HIV/AIDS Program trains mental health professionals who are currently providing services for individuals living with HIV/AIDS. The MHCPE curriculum focuses on building a knowledge base and skills in the medical, neurobehavioral, psychosocial, counseling and testing issues that may arise for mental health care providers as they care for individuals affected by HIV/AIDS. Three organizations currently provide the bulk of the training to their respective affiliates. The American Psychiatric Association provides training to psychiatrists, residents, and psychiatry medical students on the psychiatric and neuropsychiatric aspects of HIV/AIDS. The American Psychological Association primarily provides training to psychologists through their HIV Office for Psychology Education Program. This includes training in the ethics curriculum, with 10 additional HIV specific curricula. The National Association of Social Workers provides training primarily to social workers and social work trainers, focusing on triple diagnosis and adherence. In FY 2011, 3,000 persons were trained.

In FY 2011, the funding for this training program was $973,544. In FY 2012, the funding for this training program was $785,717.

Supplemental Security Income and Social Security Disability Insurance Outreach, Access and Recovery Training

The primary goal of the Supplemental Security Income (SSI) and Social Security Disability Insurance (SSDI) Outreach, Access, and Recovery (SOAR) Initiative is to train providers to develop successful SSI and SSDI applications for individuals who are homeless by increasing the quality of the disability applications and thereby reducing the decision time cycle for approvals.

In 2011, the SOAR Technical Assistance Center conducted five four-day train-the-trainer workshops in 41 states and the District of Columbia resulting in 131 new trainees. Five two-day trainings were conducted by SOAR technical assistance Center staff in four states with 140 participants. An additional 160 trainings were conducted by SOAR trainers in 40 states and the District of Columbia for a total of 4,138 participants.

In FY 2011, the funding for the SOAR training program was $2,141,668. In FY 2012, the funding for the SOAR training program was $2,355,824.

Parent Support Provider Initiative

The purpose of the National Parent Support Provider and Youth Support Specialist Initiative is to expand the children's behavioral health workforce in America. This initiative addresses the critical shortage of trained workers in the field of children's services delivery by developing core competencies and conducting workforce trainings. Certification is provided through the Certification Commission of the National Federation of Families for Children's Mental Health which requires a national exam and on-going training and supervision. In the first month of the national certification (March 2012), 70 persons applied for testing.

In FY 2011, the funding for this initiative was $150,000. No SAMHSA funds were available for FY 2012.

Child and Adolescent Psychiatry Resident Fellowship

The purpose of SAMHSA's Child and Adolescent Psychiatry Fellowship Program is to train child and adolescent psychiatry second year residents in public sector service and community- based child and adolescent psychiatry policy and practice. The fellows receive an introduction into the operation of the federal government and the American Academy of Child and Adolescent Psychiatry, including issues related to federal and state programs for children who have mental health challenges. The selected fellows have the opportunity to become involved with research, as well as to improve their writing, evaluation, and presentation abilities.

This program does not have a budget, but is supported by SAMHSA staff's time with the fellows.

National Suicide Prevention Lifeline

An objective of the National Suicide Prevention Lifeline is to increase and improve public access to crisis intervention services while promoting a consistent and evidence-informed approach to crisis hotline, chat, and text services throughout the network. Since its launch in January 2005, the Lifeline has sponsored nine Applied Suicide Intervention Skills Training (ASIST) workshops for Trainers during which 88 Lifeline centers received training. ASIST is a training program which offers a complete model of suicide first-aid intervention that provides a consistent approach to helping those contemplating suicide from initial contact through follow-up. As a result, 390 ASIST workshops have trained a total of 4,650 individuals, both professionals and volunteers alike.

In FY 2011, funding for the Lifeline training was $100,000.

Prevention Practices in School Program – Implementing the Good Behavior Game in the Nation's Disadvantaged Communities

The Prevention Practices in School initiative trains teachers and school staff to implement the Good Behavior Game (GBG) which prevents aggressive and disruptive behavior among young children in the short term and prevents antisocial behavior and the use of illicit drugs in the longer term.

Workforce development is continuous throughout the project cycle and an integral part of this program. Teachers must meet specific criteria to be considered fully trained, and the coaching models implemented in schools ensure that this is being accomplished. Training also takes place repeatedly every school year, and teachers, coaches, and project directors are able to take booster training sessions. Furthermore, specific aspects or parts of the GBG are also offered to non- teaching school staff.

At the close of the first year of the project, more than 400 coaches and teachers have been trained in GBG, and over 250 teachers are implementing GBG successfully in 21 school districts. In FY 2011, this program was funded at $735,000.

Suicide Prevention Resource Center

The Suicide Prevention Resource Center (SPRC) has been funded by SAMHSA since 2003 to provide technical assistance, training, and materials to increase the knowledge and expertise of suicide prevention practitioners and other professionals serving people at risk for suicide. SPRC also promotes collaboration among a variety of organizations that play a role in developing the field of suicide prevention. SPRC created a Provider Initiatives staff team to develop initiatives to increase the capacity of health and behavioral health care providers who can play a role in identifying and helping individuals at risk of suicide. Specifically, SPRC's Provider Initiatives aim to serve five provider groups with the potential to intervene effectively with suicidal patients: primary care, emergency departments, inpatient psychiatry, substance abuse, and mental health. SPRC's current Provider Initiatives include the following:

- *Assessing and Managing Suicide Risk: Core Competencies for Mental Health Professionals* – A one-day workshop to increase the knowledge and confidence of behavioral health professionals to work with suicidal clients and patients. Between October 2010 and the present, 4,267 social workers, psychologists, mental health counselors, psychiatrists, psychiatric nurses, and other professionals

completed Assessing and Managing Suicide Risk through workshops sponsored across the country. This total includes 1,087 professionals of the U.S. Navy.
- *Counseling on Access to Lethal Means* – An online workshop designed for providers who counsel people at risk for suicide, primarily mental health and medical providers, but also clergy and social service providers. Since the course was launched in October 2011, 364 professionals have completed the course.
- *The Suicide Prevention Toolkit for Rural Primary Care Practices* – Offered online, as a downloadable PDF, and in hard-copy. The *Toolkit,* developed by SPRC in collaboration with the Western Interstate Commission for Higher Education (WICHE), offers information and tools necessary to equip primary care settings to reduce suicide risk among their patients. The online *Toolkit* received 9,860 unique hits since October 1, 2011. SPRC staff co-led several of WICHE's in-person workshops based on the toolkit and have provided technical assistance to approximately 75 primary care practices in 20 states, including Alaska, Hawaii, Idaho, and Washington, during that time period.

In FY 2011, funding for the SPRC training program was $470,000. In FY 2012, funding for the SPRC training program was $470,000.

National Action Alliance for Suicide Prevention

The Action Alliance is a private-public collaborative advanced by SAMHSA to support implementation of the Surgeon General's National Strategy for Suicide Prevention and to increase and support both public and private efforts to reduce deaths by suicide and provide services for persons with serious thoughts of suicide. The Clinical Care and Intervention Task Force of the Action Alliance produced a report, *Suicide Care in Systems Framework,* which recommended a "whole systems" model for implementing innovative, effective suicide care in health and behavioral health populations. The Clinical Care and Intervention Task Force is working with SPRC to develop web content, materials, and technical assistance for health and behavioral health organizations wishing to adopt the leadership, systems, and workforce development required for success. Another task force, the *Clinical Workforce Preparedness Task Force,* is working to define the gaps, problems, or opportunities in training relevant to suicide prevention across all health and behavioral health professions. Research has indicated that many behavioral health professionals do not receive training in suicide risk assessment, management or treatment. The task force is in the process of assessing the current standards in the field, including assessing the presence of training standards with regard to suicide in all state licensing organizations, among health and mental health professional organizations, and in post- graduate degree programs.

Total funding for the Action Alliance was $1,000,000 in FY 2011 and $500,000 in FY 2012. This funding covered convening, educating, report production, and other costs, including staffing of the Action Alliance. Of this total, the amount spent on preparing workforce standards cannot be separated from the other expenses associated with that task force or of the overall Action Alliance.

Garrett Lee Smith Campus and State/Tribal Grantee Workforce Development Efforts

The goals of the Garrett Lee Smith (GLS) Suicide Prevention Program are: assisting communities, colleges, and universities in their efforts to prevent suicide attempts and completions, and to enhance services for youth aged 10-24, including college students with mental health and substance abuse problems that may lead to suicidal thoughts or actions. The GLS grantees use a portion of their funding to train behavioral health providers both on campuses and in the surrounding communities. Grantees provide trainers to conduct evidence- based clinical intervention programs for mental health providers; the overwhelming majority of who have not yet received professional training in assessing patients for suicidal risk or managing suicidal patients. An estimated 91,811 behavioral health care workforce persons have been trained in the GLS state and tribal program and 30,120 from the Campus program for a total of 121,931 trained. Some of the evidence-based trainings they conduct include *Assessing and Managing Suicide Risk*, *Recognizing and Responding to Suicide Risk: Essential Skills for Clinicians, Dialectical Behavioral Therapy* and *Motivational Interviewing*.

In 2011, funding for these cooperative agreements was $34,500,000. In 2012, funding for these cooperative agreements was $34,300,000. As described above, some of these funds are being used for workforce activities. However, separating out the funds used exclusively for workforce activities has not been possible to date.

Project Linking Actions for Unmet Needs in Children's Health

Project Linking Actions for Unmet Needs in Children's Health (LAUNCH) is an early childhood-focused, prevention and wellness promotion grant program, the goal of which is to ensure that all young children (birth to age 8) reach their developmental potential so that they can be successful in school and beyond. Project LAUNCH grantees work at the state, tribal and local community levels to increase coordination across child serving systems, and improve access to high quality care and evidence-based programs for young children and their families. Key to the Project LAUNCH model is workforce development activities that increase knowledge about healthy child development (particularly healthy social and emotional development) and behavioral health issues. Project LAUNCH grantees conduct a wide variety of workforce development activities with providers from multiple disciplines, including primary care providers, teachers (early education and elementary schools), home visitors, child care providers, child welfare professionals, and policymakers. Workforce development activities seek to: (1) increase knowledge of early child development, particularly social and emotional development, and children's behavioral health; (2) train providers on the appropriate use of developmental screening and assessments (including administration and interpretation); (3) train providers in evidence-based prevention practices, including individual, group, child- and family-focused interventions; and (4) help child care providers and educators to create center and classroom environments that foster healthy child development and appropriately address behavioral challenges.

In the first two and half years of the Project LAUNCH Initiative, grantees trained over 11,000 providers in 24 states and communities.

Grantees generally spend about 10-12 percent of their budgets on workforce development. Depending on the cohort (as each cohort is funded at a different level) this comes out to about $70,000–$100,000 per year/grantee. In addition, at the initiative level, the Technical Assistance Center (with an annual budget of $1.72 million) spends roughly 45 percent of its budget on training and workforce development for grantees.

In FY 2011, the approximate annual expenditure on workforce development through Project LAUNCH was about $2,700,000. In FY 2012, the approximate annual expenditure on workforce development through Project Launch was about $3,749,000.

National Child Traumatic Stress Network

Through cross-network collaborations, the National Child Traumatic Stress Network (NCTSN) groups have developed intervention approaches and associated training and dissemination products that are now being used and evaluated to improve treatment and services for children and adolescents who experience domestic and community violence, medical trauma, refugee trauma, out-of-home placement, and traumatic grief.

The NCTSN has provided over 20,000 trainings to over one million people and has developed resources for child/adolescent trauma on the NCTSN website, which receives more than 2,000 visits a day and houses over 150 Network-developed resources downloaded more than 50,000 times a year. They have developed online training in evidence-based trauma interventions, one of which has had more than 20,000 participants complete the program. A Learning Center website has also been developed that provides access to 10 expert webinars on trauma topics that have been viewed by over 7,000 individuals. In addition, the Network has developed an intensive learning collaborative model for service providers and conducted 17 of these learning collaboratives for more than 800 service providers.

In FY 2011 and FY 2012, the funding for NCTSN grantees to conduct provider training and other workforce development activities was approximately $10,000,000 per year.

Center for Promoting Alternatives to Seclusion and Restraint Through Trauma-Informed Approaches and the National Center for Trauma Informed Care

The purpose of this Center is to provide national leadership in reducing the pervasive, harmful, and costly health impact of violence and trauma by integrating trauma-informed approaches throughout health and behavioral health systems, and to divert people with substance abuse and mental health disorders from criminal and juvenile justice systems into trauma-informed treatment, supports, and recovery. The goals for the Center are to expand the use of trauma- informed practices to end the use of seclusion, restraint, and other coercive practices. The contract tasks provide for the development of a structured learning process to be used in implementation of trauma informed care in a collaborative and integrated manner that integrates consumer/ survivor voice and leadership, including training, virtual training, remote and on-site technical assistance, meeting logistics, product development, process evaluation, and knowledge dissemination.

In 2012, the Center completed 157 training/technical assistance events. Forty-one events focused principally on trauma-informed practices and 116 focused on the reduction of seclusion and restraint through trauma-informed practices. Many requests involved multiple systems, and project staff work with applicants to encourage collaboration and cross-systems training whenever possible. Approximately 10,000 people received training/technical assistance through this contract since 2010. In addition to the trainings, four webinars were conducted. The Center also produced a number of products including reports, issue briefs and guides, and have convened conferences focused on the use of peers to prevent the use of seclusion and restraints and implementing trauma informed care in services systems.

The budget for the Center for FY 2011 was $2,477,198. The FY 2012 budget was $2,612,681.

SAMHSA GAINS Center for Behavioral Health and Justice Transformation

The SAMHSA GAINS Center's primary focus is on expanding access to community-based services for adults diagnosed with co-occurring mental illness and substance use disorders at all points of contact with the justice system. The SAMHSA GAINS Center developed curricula to train criminal justice professionals to understand the impact of trauma on men and women with serious mental illness and to improve safety by learning new ways to interact with people who are traumatized. The training is targeted to police, community corrections (probation, parole, and pre-trial service officers), and court personnel (judges, attorneys, case managers and treatment providers). Over the past 12 months, 350 people have been trained in 10 cities. The program also includes a train-the-trainer curriculum that focuses on justice specific community service providers, court administrators, court deputies, district and assistant district attorneys, judges, probation officers, re-entry staff, treatment court coordinators, forensic or clinical caseworkers, community service boards, and state mental health and substance abuse agencies. In February 2012, a day and a half train-the-trainer event was held for 36 individuals including community service providers, court administrators, court deputies, district and assistant district attorneys, judges, probation officers, re-entry staff, treatment court coordinators, forensic or clinical caseworkers, community service boards, and state behavioral health agencies.

In FY 2011, funding for the GAINS Center training program was $70,000. In FY 2012, funding for the GAINS Center training program was $70,000.

Bringing Recovery Support Services to Scale – Technical Assistance Center Services

The Bringing Recovery Supports to Scale Technical Assistance Center Strategy (BRSS TACS) contract meets a major need to identify effective approaches to develop and sustain behavioral health care recovery support initiatives in states and systems across the nation. Specifically, it will provide policy and practice guidelines and information and technical assistance to states, systems, providers, and others to assist in transforming behavioral health services.

This project intends to support the expansion and integration of recovery supports via the development and operation of a Resource Center on Recovery Supports. This will be accomplished through three main tasks – policy and practice analyses, training and education, and technical assistance. The Resource Center is a partnership among people in recovery from addictions who have experience working in the addictions recovery field and people in recovery from mental health problems and conditions and/or serious emotional disabilities who have experience working in the mental health consumer field, as well as people with co-occurring disorders, trauma, and a variety of allies, supporters, and other stakeholders in recovery-oriented services and systems.

As part of SAMHSA's BRSS TACS initiative, SAMHSA hosted an Expert Panel on the provision of peer recovery support services which included components specifically focused on the development of Recovery Coaches/Peer Specialists. One outcome of this effort is to develop guidelines for States working with Recovery Coaches and Peer Specialists working with both the mental health and addictions recovery populations.

In FY 2011, this effort totaled approximately $50,000. In FY 2012, this effort totaled approximately $50,000.

The National Network to Eliminate Disparities in Behavioral Health

In 2008, SAMHSA established the National Network to Eliminate Disparities in Behavioral Health (NNED) to promote workforce development for community-based behavioral health organizations that serve diverse racial, ethnic and sexual minority communities.

These organizations often have limited resources for and access to training for their staff. The NNED, a virtual network of these community-based provider organizations, provides the following opportunities to advance the capacity and strengthen the quality of this workforce:

- *Best practices in implementation science* – NNEDLearn provides six training tracks on selected evidence-based and culturally adapted practices. These are practices that have been selected by the NNED membership. Participants in these tracks convene with a master trainer for a two-day training, and continue with six months of regular follow-up coaching to support implementation of the newly acquired practice. Examples of training tracks include Motivational Interviewing, Culturally Adapted Cognitive Behavioral Therapy for Latinos, Empowering Our Spirit Suicide Prevention for Tribes, and Strengthening Families, Seeking Safety. In the past two years of the NNEDLearn training, 250 participants representing over 45 community-based organizations have participated in this intensive, skill-building training.
- *Virtual Communities of Practice* – Training on a specific practice through webinars, teleconferences and a virtual online "office space" and discussion forum. Each Communities of Practice (CoP) is led by an expert trainer or developer of the practice. Examples of interventions addressed in these CoPs include Project Venture (an evidenced-based substance abuse prevention practice for tribal youth), Multi-Family Group Treatment for Latino Families, and Bienvenido – A Mental Health Promotion for Latino Immigrants. Nine CoPs have been offered, serving over 150 practitioners from community-based behavioral health organizations.
- *NNEDShare* – A repository of emerging and innovative interventions geared to improving outreach, engagement, practice and outcomes for diverse cultural populations. This is a searchable database on the NNED website that promotes cross-agency sharing and peer-to-peer training and technical assistance. The NNED has been effective in bringing workforce training opportunities and in–language training to diverse community-based organizations.

Evidence-based and community-culturally based practices have been shared and collaborations built among the participants in the NNED, toward the goal of advancing quality care for these communities. Since 2008, the NNED has grown from 35 to 534 community-based organizations in 2012.

In both FY 2011 and 2012, the NNED initiative was funded at $625,000. This activity is funded out of the agency overhead funds, consistent with our 501(d)(3) authority. The 501(d)(3) authority allows SAMHSA to tap programs to "carry out administrative and financial management, policy development & planning....functions."

Provider Business Operations Contract

In light of coming changes brought by the opportunities of the Affordable Care Act, SAMHSA is undertaking a special effort to train and develop learning collaboratives for providers serving persons with behavioral health needs in a specialty setting. This effort will assist providers with business planning, compliance requirements, use of HIT, billing requirements, and the process of being part of a provider network for an insurance company. Without this help, many specialty providers will not be ready to move into the world of provider networks that are part of Qualified Health Plans and increasing managed care in Medicaid and employer-based insurance mechanisms. Furthermore, the number of available specialty providers serving persons with more extensive addiction and mental health needs will decline below already unacceptable levels.

FY 2012 funding for this effort includes $1,627,972. This activity is funded out of the agency overhead funds, consistent with our 501(d)(3) authority. The 501(d)(3) authority allows SAMHSA to tap programs to "carry out administrative and financial management, policy development & planning....functions."

HRSA Behavioral Health Workforce Programs

HRSA recognizes the importance of behavioral health and the links among mental, physical and emotional wellbeing. This is reflected across HRSA's broad portfolio of programs and services. HRSA promotes integrated behavioral health service delivery in primary care settings and effective referral arrangements, when indicated, to specialty behavioral health provider organizations.

Delivering mental health and addiction services in primary care settings helps to reduce the prejudice and discrimination often experienced by persons with mental health or substance abuse problems. Serving people with behavioral health concerns in collaborative primary care settings supports a "no wrong door" approach to care.

The framework HRSA uses is built on efforts to position primary care within the broader context of community health, to align primary care and behavioral health seamlessly, and to consistently build relationships with stakeholders to improve the delivery and access of health and behavioral health services to vulnerable populations. Examples of HRSA programs focusing on behavioral health include the following.

Health Centers

The Affordable Care Act makes a major investment in Health Centers expanding and strengthening these providers. Today these centers operate 8,500 clinics across the country, serving over 20 million patients regardless of their ability to pay. Two-thirds of health centers provide mental health treatment or counseling services, and one-third provides substance abuse counseling and treatment. According to health center data, depression is among the top ten primary reasons that patients visit a health center.

These services are provided in large part through over 5,000 FTE behavioral health providers in health centers. This includes more than 400 psychologists, 400 psychiatrists, nearly 1,400 licensed clinical social workers, 1,000 licensed mental health counselors, and 875 substance use disorder treatment providers. HRSA provides training and resources for these professionals and for the primary care professionals to increase their knowledge and skills about the prevention and treatment of mental and substance use disorders.

HRSA encourages its health center grantees to include the SBIRT approach; and SBIRT is now a service indicated on the yearly health center data reporting system that HRSA administers.

HRSA Workforce Specific Programs

Strengthening the behavioral health workforce is a critically important component of HRSA's overall efforts to expand the nation's health care workforce. HRSA's National Health Service Corps, which also received strong support through the Affordable Care Act, are health professionals who provide primary health care services in underserved communities in exchange for either loan repayment assistance or scholarships to help pay the costs of their medical education. With investments from the Affordable Care Act, the Corps had over 9,908 health professionals serving in underserved communities in 2012.

In 1995, when psychologists, social workers, psychiatrists and other behavioral health providers were first admitted to the Corps, there were exactly *five awardees*. As of September 2012, roughly three out of 10 NHSC clinicians in the field are primary care mental health or substance abuse practitioners for a total of 2,809 practitioners in the following disciplines:

psychiatrists, clinical psychologists, clinical social workers, licensed professional counselors, marriage and family therapists, and psychiatric nurse specialists. NHSC mental and behavioral health practitioners may provide substance abuse treatment.

HRSA also supports the Graduate Psychology Education Program which provides grants to train psychologists working with underserved populations. For academic year 2010-2011, there were 710 trainees, of which 416 (58 percent) served in medically underserved communities.

HRSA has a new Mental and Behavioral Health Education and Training Grants Program that aims to increase the number of social workers and psychologists who pursue clinical work with high-need and high-demand populations. As a result of this funding, accredited graduate social work schools and accredited psychology schools will be able to increase their overall number of enrolled students, create more field placement and internship slots for students, and ultimately increase the number of clinical providers working with underserved populations. These professionals may work with individuals with mental illness, with substance use disorders, or with both.

HRSA's Veterans' Mental Health Project was created to address the post-deployment mental health and substance abuse issues of veterans and their families through the training of primary care providers across the nation.

SAMHSA - HRSA Workforce Collaborative Initiatives

Implementation of the Affordable Care Act will require an expanded and appropriately trained workforce. Many of the authorized workforce activities were delegated to HRSA for implementation either through the expansion of existing programs or new authorizations. To better integrate the delivery of behavioral health and primary care in this new environment, SAMHSA and HRSA began a number of collaborative efforts to enhance the workforce. Some of these activities are supported through a formal IAA, while others reflect a more informal emphasis on data analysis, model development for integrated primary and behavioral health care, technical assistance for integrated programs or those wishing to develop integrated approaches, information sharing, joint training, and other collaborative efforts.

Center for Integrated Health Solutions

SAMHSA and HRSA are jointly funding a national resource center that provides training and technical assistance to community behavioral health programs, community health centers, and other primary care organizations. The resource center helps develop models of integrated care across behavioral health and primary care. This effort recognizes the increasing role primary care plays in screening, preventing and treating mental health and substance abuse problems, and the need for persons with serious mental illness to have their primary health care needs addressed in the same setting where they receive care for the mental health condition(s).

The CIHS provides training and technical assistance on the bi-directional integration of primary and behavioral health care and related workforce development. The CIHS provides training and technical assistance to the currently funded 64 community behavioral health organizations that have SAMHSA Primary and Behavioral Health Care Integration (PBHCI) grants as well as to community health centers and other primary care and behavioral health organizations.

The CIHS has engaged in a wide array of activities that impact the full continuum of workforce communities under PBHCI. Some of the highlights are below.

Curriculum Development
- Psychiatrist Training Curriculum – Developed a 6 Module Psychiatrist Curriculum designed to increase psychiatrists' capacity to practice and/or consult in integrated health settings.
    - Module 1: Introduction to Primary Care Consultation Psychiatry
    - Module 2: Building a Collaborative Care Team
    - Module 3: Psychiatrist Consulting in Primary Care
    - Module 4: Behavioral Health in Primary Care
    - Module 5: Medical Patients with Psychiatric Illness
    - Module 6: The role of the Psychiatrist in the Public Mental Health System.
- Whole Health Action Management – Developed a national curriculum and pilot tested the curriculum with consumers and staff representatives from 50 out of 56 SAMHSA PBHCI grantees. The program creates workforce capacity by preparing consumers to serve as health educators and coaches. The two-day *Whole Health Action Management Peer Support Training* guides participants through a person-centered planning process to set a whole health and resiliency

goal. Once the goal is set, the participant guide shifts to creating and self-managing new health behavior by implementing an eight-week whole health peer support group that engages in a weekly action plan for success. The training is designed to support the emerging peer workforce to move into new health integration service models like health homes.
- Primary Care Physician Training Curriculum – Developed a Primary Care Physician Training Curriculum designed to create capacity for primary care physicians to treat and support individuals with a serious mental illness. Prevalence, Serious Mental iIllness Characteristics, Pharmacological and Behavioral Interventions are highlighted.
  - Module 1: Working with Patients with a Severe and Persistent Mental Illness; What Should Primary Care Physicians Know?
  - Module 2: Update on Psychopharmacology for Primary Care Physicians; Depression and Anxiety Part I & II.
- Masters Level Social Work Competency-Based Curriculum – The Integrated Healthcare Curriculum for Schools of Social Works is a competency-based curriculum to prepare Masters of Social Work students for behavioral health practice focused on integrative and collaborative primary-behavioral health care. The curriculum will prepare future Masters level social workers to enter the workforce with the needed competencies to provide and lead integrated health care.

Trainings
- Health Navigator/Care Management Training – The Health Navigator/Care Management training program is designed to transform traditional mental health case management programs into assuming responsibility for the whole health of the individuals they serve. The day-long training covers a variety of topics related to a new and broader knowledge base for case managers. The program conducted seven, two-day Health Navigator Trainings for SAMHSA PBHCI grantee organizations.
- Mental Health First Aid Training – Mental Health First Aid (MHFA) is a public education program that creates capacity within communities to identify, understand, and respond to signs of mental illnesses and substance use disorders. MHFA introduces individual participants to risk factors and warning signs of mental health problems and substance use disorders, builds understanding of their

impact, and overviews common treatments. Those who take the 12-hour course to certify as Mental Health First Aiders learn a five-step action plan encompassing the skills, resources and knowledge to help an individual in crisis connect with appropriate professional, peer, social, and self-help care.
- Trained five rural health centers in MHFA.
- MHFA training for federal staff.
- Provided statewide Primary Care Association training to Northwest Region for 25 FQHCs.
- Provided MHFA Training for three federal agencies.
- Completed a Spanish translation of MHFA.
• Suicide Prevention Training for Primary Care Practices – This training is targeted to increasing the capacity of primary care practitioners and behavioral health professionals who work in or frequently collaborate with primary care, rural providers, FQHC's, and residency programs in family medicine to identify and intervene with those at risk of suicide. Seventy-six percent of individuals who die by suicide had contact with their primary care practitioners in the month prior to their suicide. The training supports the implementation of state-of-the-art suicide prevention practices while minimizing the disruption of normal operations. The training is tailored to meet the needs of the primary care site or educational center. CIHS conducted four trainings in rural communities.
• Integrated Care Conference Track – The NACHC developed an integrated care track for FQHC on the importance of Integrated Healthcare and factors they could consider when training their workforce.

Integrated Health & Wellness Training Scholarships
- Cherokee Integrated Health Model – CIHS provided two scholarships for SAMHSA PBHCI Grantee teams to visit Cherokee Health Systems to learn from integrated treatment team approaches.
- University of Massachusetts Certificate Program in Primary Care Behavioral Health – CIHS provided scholarships for up to 80 individuals from PBHCI grantee organizations the opportunity to participate in the Certificate Program in Primary Care Behavioral Health provided by the University of Massachusetts Medical School.
- University of Colorado Denver Tobacco Cessation and Wellness Program – CIHS contracted with the University of Colorado Tobacco

Cessation and Wellness Program to develop an assessment tool to provide direct technical assistance. The assessment tool is being piloted with SAMHSA PBHCI grantees.

Stakeholder Meeting
- Workforce Issues: Integrating Substance Abuse Services into Primary Care Summit – CIHS provided technical and logistical support to the White House Office of National Drug Control Policy, SAMHSA, and HRSA hosted event about *Workforce Issues: Integrating Substance Abuse Services into Primary Care Summit* on August 10-11, 2011. Deliverables included Meeting Planning, Workforce Report, Presentation, and Summit Summary Report.

Workforce Webinars

CIHS conducts various webinars targeted towards different workforce areas, for example:

- Sharing of information in an electronic environment.
- Specific confidentiality and consent law and regulations for certain substance abuse treatment records (42 CFR Part 2).
- Motivational Interviewing.
- The role and practice of peer supports.
- National Health Service Corp (NHSC).
- InSHAPE approach to wellness for individuals with a serious mental illness.
- Short-term behavioral health interventions in primary care.
- Smoking cessation, for practitioners working in FQHCs.

Products
- Accessing the National Health Service Corp: A Guide for Community Behavioral Health Providers and Primary Care Partners – This guide assists behavioral health sites in becoming NHSC-approved sites and expanding the behavioral health workforce in those communities. The guide includes opportunities to recruit practitioners and clinicians interested in NHSC employment and an overview of the NHSC loan repayment benefits.
- CIHS Workforce Guiding Principles – This document is a compilation of areas and characteristics that organizations implementing integrated

health strategies can use to guide the development of workforce strategic plans.
- Workforce Resource Inventory – This inventory is a compilation of workforce resources (trainings, articles, literature, tools) related to integrated primary and behavioral health care.
- Gap Analysis of Integrated Health Workforce – This analysis is a review and synthesis of existing literature and resources related to integrated primary and behavioral health workforce to identify gaps and develop recommendations for future initiatives.
- Peer Roadmap – This product outlines the states that have incorporated a definition for the use of peers for the delivery of services within their Medicaid State Plan.

In FY 2011, funding for this cooperative agreement was $350,000 from HRSA and $5 million from SAMHSA's PBHCI program funding As described above, funds are being used for workforce activities; however, separating out the funds specific to workforce development activities has not been possible, as many activities support grantees, develop workforce, provide training, and produce and disseminate materials at once.

In FY 2012, the funding from SAMHSA for this Center was limited by Congressional Appropriations to $2,000,000, and now supports only SAMHSA grantees. HRSA continued to contribute $365,000 for this joint effort allowing CIHS to maintain a broader impact within the limits of available funding.

SAMHSA and HRSA Behavioral Health Minimum Data Set Project

As has been referenced in this report, the lack of any national database or information on the addiction services and mental health workforce is a major hindrance in identifying and remedying issues.

In 2011, SAMHSA entered into an IAA with HRSA to ensure the inclusion of the behavioral health workforce in HRSA's development of a Minimum Data Set (MDS) for the health care workforce. The purpose of this IAA is to:

- Develop guidelines for minimum data sets;
- Support and assist stakeholders with the collection of behavioral health professions data;
- Provide technical assistance and resources to enhance stakeholder data collection efforts;

- Build a national behavioral health workforce dataset; and
- Identify possible methods for providing federal agencies access to such data.

In order to accomplish the objectives of this project, HRSA and SAMHSA are identifying which occupations to include in the behavioral health workforce database, data sources, and what data are being collected; developing the questionnaire to be used; identifying the organizations in each chosen behavioral health care profession that are best able to implement the MDS; and recruiting these organizations to participate in the MDS.

This is a one-year project that is underway, with HRSA's National Center for Healthcare Workforce Analysis taking the lead. SAMHSA and HRSA are working closely together, with SAMHSA staff providing subject matter expertise to HRSA staff that provides oversight and management of the project.

In FY 2011, the budget for this project was $500,000. No SAMHSA funds were available for FY 2012.

Military Culture Training

The purpose of the IAA is to facilitate cooperative efforts between SAMHSA and HRSA, Bureau of Health Professions in order to provide technical assistance, competency and curriculum development, continuing education, and related evaluation to the primary care and education field related to the mental and behavioral health and substance abuse issues of veterans and their families.

SAMHSA provides technical consultation on the mental and behavioral health and substance abuse needs of veterans and their families to the project team, as requested, and provides necessary feedback, review, and comment to HRSA in order to provide technical direction to the contractor. HRSA through the National AHEC Organization (NAO) provides technical assistance to the primary care and education workforce focused on the mental and substance abuse issues of veterans and their families to include curriculum development and inter- professional continuing education for health care providers on the mental and substance abuse issues of veterans and their families. In addition, the NAO will evaluate the effect of the continuing education curriculum/courses on the practice of participating health care providers. SAMHSA provided $500,000 in FY 2011 to support this effort. No SAMHSA funds were available for FY 2012.

Other SAMHSA/HRSA Collaborations

Given the importance of workforce issues, SAMHSA and HRSA are working to optimize the potential to collaborate, maximizing the efficiency of authorized and appropriated funds. Examples of such collaborations include HRSA's request for SAMHSA's assistance on the selection of behavioral health training and speakers for the NHSC Awardee conferences, which are conducted several times a year for those in the loan repayment program. The topics are reviewed annually and are selected based on the needs expressed by the conference attendees and the evidence-based practices that are available.

Another example is the coordination of education and training opportunities in HBCUs through the respective contracts that SAMHSA and HRSA have with the Morehouse School of Medicine. Though only just begun, the goal of this collaboration is to foster more cross-training that would enhance integration and provide expanded audiences for the offerings from each of these centers.

SAMHSA and HRSA are also identifying information and materials available from SAMHSA needed by HRSA funded community health centers to make those resources available to practitioners in those settings.

SAMHSA and HRSA are also working with other HHS agencies and offices to develop training for community health workers on the use of SBIRT. This training will be conducted in collaboration with the Department of Labor and through a HRSA-funded AHEC provider, with funding from HRSA, SAMHSA and the Office of Assistant Secretary for Health.

SAMHSA/HRSA Joint Listening Session

Recognizing the importance of the behavioral health workforce, SAMHSA and HRSA jointly hosted a listening session for behavioral health stakeholders on June 5, 2012, specifically to discuss and identify behavioral health workforce issues and approaches to addressing them.[5]

The joint listening session focused on four behavioral health workforce areas: (1) capacity; (2) data; (3) training and education; and (4) the non-traditional workforce. This summary incorporates the major themes that SAMHSA and HRSA heard during this listening session, as well as written comments received after the meeting. SAMHSA and HRSA thank those in attendance, both in person and by teleconference, for their involvement and efforts on workforce issues, and also those who took the time to provide additional written comments.

Behavioral Health Workforce Capacity

Increasing the behavioral health workforce capacity was a major area of concern and the themes from the discussants included:

- Continue to build behavioral health workforce capacity through the NHSC.
- Develop, recruit and support for behavioral health professions at all educational levels.
- Improve professional training through development of more internship placements in safety net provider locations, such as health centers, and provide direct student support for education through scholarships and loan repayment.
- Encourage the use of technology to expand the reach to clinicians, such as use of Internet capabilities for therapies, while ensuring clear standards and monitoring of professionals to assure public protection.
- Modeled on the SAMHSA-HRSA CIHS, expand efforts to provide professional cross training of staff in both primary and behavioral health care to promote integrated care for persons with mental health or addiction problems.
- Recruit potential workers earlier in the educational pipeline to encourage interest in behavioral health careers.
- Promote development of career development pathways, especially for substance abuse counselors.
- Identify and address the state credentialing and licensure issues that make it increasingly difficult for those with lower level licenses to bill independently in insurance-based payment systems.
- Address inadequate payment issues for services performed by community mental health and substance abuse centers.

Data Needs and Collection Processes

Several of the attendees expressed enthusiasm for the current SAMHSA-HRSA MDS initiative and recommended:

- Continue support to develop the MDS for behavioral health professionals as it will provide core, consistent, and continuous data on demographics, practices, and settings.
- Review current public and professional association data collection efforts to see what workforce elements they contain that could be incorporated into the MDS.

Training and Education Needs

A number of key themes arose during this part of the listening session including:

- Increase efforts to train the workforce in cultural diversity (including lesbian, gay, bisexual, and transgender [LGBT] issues) and promote internship training in culturally diverse settings.
- Expand pre-professional efforts such as cross-training of behavioral staff and primary care staff regarding integrated care and disseminate information on how to develop effective multidisciplinary primary and behavioral health teams.
- Encourage the incorporation of technology to more effectively deliver training and education.
- Promote training on motivational interviewing and other evidence-based practices for behavioral health services.
- Foster effective methods of teaching evidence-based practices to increase adoption in the field, such as greater use of clinical supervision and applied continuing education programs.
- Encourage the inclusion of peers, persons in recovery, mental health consumers, and family members in professional education and training programs and in research programs that identify evidence-based practices.
- Assist providers and persons in recovery to develop and capture practice-based evidence to identify effective and emerging practices.
- Prepare primary and behavioral health safety net professionals to successfully join provider networks of managed behavioral health organizations.

Non-Traditional Workforce

Comments on the growth and greater use of the non-traditional workforce related to such issues as the need for appropriate training and education, as well as increased treatment capacity. The non-traditional workforce needs to be included in data collection efforts, including those in recovery from mental and substance use conditions, as well as community health workers, patient navigators, and health educators. Additional recommendations included:

- Continue to support the clarification of needed competencies for peers and family members; encourage creation of a peer professional career ladder, including training and supervision of peers by peers.
- Collect and disseminate information on state-specific descriptions of peer services for Medicaid programs and other insurers, including: identification of peer services that are reimbursed; descriptions of coverage limitations or specific supervision or training requirements; payment mechanisms and rates; and how to encourage the greater inclusion of peers in integrated health care teams.
- Encourage funding of innovations and services that include peers in accountable care and other alternative payment programs, as well as in block grant and competitive grant programs where possible.
- Build bridges between peer counselors, health educators, and community health workers in primary care settings; encourage their participation in prevention and wellness issues as well as programs or activities that help people maintain their recovery.
- Include peers as navigators and enrollment/eligibility assistants in state and federally facilitated health insurance marketplaces and in Medicaid expansion programs.
- Work with community colleges to develop curriculum and supports for peer and other alternative practitioners to assist licensed behavioral health practitioners.

CONCLUSION

The behavioral health workforce in the United States is dedicated, passionate and capable. Whether conducting prevention activities or services; serving persons with addictions, persons with mental illness, persons with both, or their families; or supporting people in recovery, they are without question a small but mighty force working to protect, maintain and improve the health of America. Yet, as a whole, the workforce is too few, aging into retirement, inadequately reimbursed; inadequately supported and trained, and facing significant changes affecting practice, credentialing, funding, and ability to keep up with changes in practice models driven by changing science, technologies and systems. Additionally, the aging of the population, the many new veterans with behavioral health needs and individuals with new access to coverage making it possible for them to get treatment for their addiction and/or mental illness will strain the already overtaxed workforce. Prevention, treatment and recovery supports will not be available, if there are not sufficient numbers of adequately trained preventionists, mental health and addictions professionals, and licensed or certified peer and alternative providers.

While SAMHSA and HRSA, as federal agencies, collaborate extensively and have significant programs and activities to train and support new and existing providers, each is limited by its authorities and its funding in what they can do to address the critical issues.

The issue of workforce development in the behavioral health field has long been a critical one. Recent moves in the behavioral health care field toward services integration along with the passage of health reform legislation have further heightened the need for the development of a well-trained, highly skilled, diverse and productive workforce. Now, more than ever, the scarcity of strong, standardized data on the workforce poses itself as an issue to be addressed. SAMHSA and HRSA will continue to include this significant issue in their strategic planning and programming to the extent their authorities and funding allow. They will also continue their collaborative efforts with each other and with other federal partners to ensure that the needs of the addiction and mental health workforce are identified and at the forefront as other health care workforce issues are discussed and addressed.

APPENDIX A. EXAMPLES OF SAMHSA-HRSA ACTIVITIES RELATED TO BEHAVIORAL HEALTH WORKFORCE – LISTENING SESSION SUMMARY

On June 5, 2012, the Substance Abuse and Mental Health Services Administration (SAMHSA) and the Health Resources and Services Administration (HRSA) hosted a listening session with stakeholders that focused on four behavioral health workforce areas: capacity, data, training and education, and the non-traditional workforce. The thoughtful input, both at the meeting and in correspondence, is being considered as both agencies move forward with program plans. To assist in understanding SAMHSA and HRSA workforce activities already underway, the following summary of current SAMHSA and HRSA activities was developed.

Behavioral Health Workforce Capacity

Overall Capacity

The Mental and Behavioral Health Education and Training Grants (MBHETG) Program: HRSA has awarded 24 accredited social work and psychology programs with 3-year funding. The MBHETG program encourages education and training addressing the behavioral health needs of high-need and high-demand populations by: (1) increasing the number of enrolled graduate social work and psychology students; and (2) creating more internship and field placement slots to increase the number of knowledgeable clinical providers working with high- need and high-demand populations.

National Health Services Corps (NHSC): HRSA's NHSC builds healthy communities by strengthening the health care workforce and continues to support individuals in behavioral and mental disciplines and practices/sites. The SAMHSA-HRSA Center for Integrated Health Solutions (CIHS) has developed a guide to assist behavioral health sites in understanding the NHSC and the process for becoming an approved NHSC site (see http://www.integration.samhsa.gov/sliders/NHSC_doc.pdf).

Advanced nursing educational efforts include behavioral health: HRSA's Advanced Education Nursing Traineeship (AENT) supports traineeships for primary care Nurse Practitioners (NP), some of which are psychiatric/mental health NPs. The Advanced Nursing Education (ANE) program and the Nurse Education, Practice, Quality, and Retention (NEPQR) program promote interprofessional education with behavioral health social workers.

Integrated Primary Care and Behavioral Care Workforce

Integrated Summit: In August 2011, ONDCP, HRSA, and SAMHSA sponsored the "Workforce Issues: Integrating Substance Abuse Services into Primary Care Summit." Identified workforce needs included: increasing addictions training in primary care professional's curricula, the necessity for career ladders and greater role definitions between primary care and behavioral health specialists.

Graduate Psychology Education (GPE) Program: HRSA grants in the GPE program support interdisciplinary training for health service psychologists to provide mental and behavioral health care services to underserved populations, such as those in rural areas, older adults, children, chronically ill or disabled persons, and victims of abuse or trauma, including returning military personnel.

Geriatric Training for Physicians, Dentists, and Behavioral and Mental Health Professionals Program: The Geriatric Training for Physicians, Dentists, and Behavioral and Mental Health Professionals Program supports 1-year faculty retraining and 2-year fellowship programs to assist physicians, dentists, and behavioral and mental health professionals who teach or plan to teach geriatric medicine, geriatric dentistry, or geriatric behavioral and mental health. The program supports learning on caring for elderly people at different levels of wellness and functioning. It provides training with elderly from diverse socioeconomic, racial, and ethnic backgrounds in a range of services, such as geriatric consultation, acute care, dental care, psychiatry, day and home care, rehabilitation, extended care, ambulatory care, and community care for older people with mental retardation.

Integrated Primary Care and Behavioral Care in the Workforce

Integrated Summit: In August 2011, the White House Office of National Drug Control Policy, HRSA, and SAMHSA sponsored the "Workforce Issues: Integrating Substance Abuse Services into Primary Care Summit." The summit identified many workforce needs, including: increasing addictions training in primary care professional's curricula, the necessity for career ladders, and a greater role for definitions between primary care and behavioral health specialists.

Multidisciplinary training includes behavioral health under Area Health Education Centers (AHECs): HRSA's AHEC grantees (i.e., medical schools, nursing schools, and health sciences centers) organize interdisciplinary and inter-professional training involving psychologists and other behavioral health professionals as practicable. Specific behavioral health topics include motivational interviewing, other evidence-based practices, and inclusion of peers/consumers in education and training.

Regional workforce training: SAMHSA's Addiction Technology Transfer Centers (ATTCs) accelerate lasting change in behavioral health care systems by translating, disseminating and promoting the adoption and implementation of effective and culturally-sensitive clinical practices. They offer distance education productions and workforce development. In addition to providing region-specific training and systems change efforts, the ATTC Network has areas of national focus that include leadership institutes and collaboration with the National Institute on Drug Abuse (NIDA) to develop products and promote the adoption of evidence-based practices.

Behavioral health workforce in health centers: HRSA's Bureau of Primary Health Care (BPHC) is working through the SAMHSA-HRSA CIHS to build workforce capacity across health centers with limited behavioral health capacity through the provision of training and technical assistance on integrated care.

Cross Training between Primary Care and Behavioral Care

Training in pain management for prescribing physicians, nurses and dentists: SAMHSA supports face-to-face and online continuing medical education (CME) courses, entitled *Prescribing Opioids for Chronic Pain: Balancing Safety & Efficacy*, on safe opioid prescribing for chronic pain for primary care physicians, oral surgeons, advanced practice nurses, and physician assistants.

Training physicians for prescribing buprenorphine: Through the Prescribers Clinical Support System for Buprenorphine (PCSS-B), SAMHSA offers the eight hour training required to apply for a buprenorphine waiver required to prescribing privileges. The training is a combination of CD-based training and face-to-face training.

Screening, Brief Intervention and Referral to Treatment (SBIRT) Medical Residency Training: SAMHSA supports the SBIRT Medical Residency Training grants, designed to train the next generation of physicians in SBIRT practice. This program includes curriculum development and training for current residents and the primary care community in SBIRT practices.

Psychologists in Health Centers: In July 2011, HRSA's BPHC hosted a grantee training specific to the hiring of psychologists at health centers: "The Value of Psychologists in Health Centers." Topics covered included current statistics on psychologists in health centers and how integrated service increases financial outcomes and quality of care; improves clinical staff recruitment and retention; and provides other benefits for the health centers.

Pipeline Activities for Behavioral Health Professions

The Health Careers Opportunity Program (HCOP): HRSA's HCOP exposes students throughout the educational pipeline to a wide array of health careers, including careers in behavioral health. The grantees provide academic enhancement, structured summer programming in health centers, academic health careers clubs and grade- specific curriculum.

NHSC pipeline activity: HRSA's NHSC attended the National Association of Student Financial Aid Administrators National Conference in Chicago in July 2012 and will generate awareness amongst financial aid administrators, including those in the mental and behavioral health field.

AHEC pipeline activities: HRSA's AHEC grantees provided health career training and/or academic enhancement experiences to 9-12th graders that included behavioral health careers. Emphasis is placed on outreach to underrepresented minority populations, educationally or economically disadvantaged individuals, and/or rural populations.

Workforce Diversity and Career Ladders

National Network for the Elimination of Disparities in Behavioral Health (NNED): SAMHSA's NNED works to increase capacities to address the behavioral health care needs of racially and ethnically diverse populations.

Center for Excellence in Historically Black Colleges: SAMHSA's cooperative agreement with Historically Black Colleges and Universities supports a Center for Excellence in Substance Abuse and Mental Health which provides student internships at minority serving institutions.

The Minority Fellowship Program (MFP): SAMHSA's MFP provides funding to oversee the fellowship opportunities to behavioral health professionals that encourage doctoral and post-doctoral development of nurses, psychiatrists, social workers, psychologists, marriage and family therapists, and professional counselors.

Addictions counselor pathways: SAMHSA supported the development of pathways for the addictions counseling profession, which can serve as a model to assist providers in staff retention.

Data Needs and Collection Processes

Minimum Data Set (MDS) on behavioral health professionals: The HRSA National Center for Health Workforce Analysis, in collaboration with SAMHSA, is actively developing a Minimum Data Set (MDS) to collect more information on the core behavioral health professions. Current efforts are focused on engaging multiple behavioral health professional organizations in convening meetings to review the necessary data elements for a survey instrument in their field. The professions currently involved include psychiatrists, psychologists, social workers, licensed professional counselors, and substance abuse counselors.

Training and Education Needs

Culturally Competent and Special Populations Training

Cultural, including LGBT, training: HRSA's HIV/AIDS Bureau (HAB), through AIDS Education and Training Centers (AETCs), provides training to the workforce on cultural diversity. From July 2010 through June 2011, over 4,000 behavioral health professionals attended one or more training events sponsored by AETCs.

Health center training on LGBT issues: HRSA's BPHC has a national cooperative agreement for the National LGBT Health Education Center to help community health centers improve the health of LGBT populations. The Center has conducted national and local trainings, and provided consultations with health centers, many of which include behavioral health professionals.

Substance abuse treatment providers on LGBT issues: SAMHSA's ATTC Network has developed a curriculum for substance abuse providers on treating LGBT individuals with substance use disorders.

Training in behavioral health in geriatrics training: HRSA has four programs that provide geriatric training and education that include mental health and substance abuse issues. These programs provide education and training in the areas health problems of the elderly and their caregivers including mental health and substance abuse problems.

Emergency preparedness for elders: In 2006, HRSA's Geriatric Education Centers received the SAMHSA-supported curricula developed by the *Annapolis Coalition on the Behavioral Health Workforce* on emergency preparedness for behavioral health professionals working with the elderly. This curricula continues to be revised and updated to reflect the latest research and information and is used both nationally and internationally.

Hiring veterans at health centers: HRSA has partnered with the National Association of Community Health Centers (NACHC) to assist veterans in obtaining jobs with health centers around the country.

Training for Evidence-Based Practices

Training for physicians, dentists and others prescribing opioid therapies: SAMHSA has two efforts providing training for prescribers: Opioid Therapies (PCSS-O) and Buprenorphine (PCSS-B) grants. The PCSS-O assists physicians, dentists and other medical professionals in the appropriate use of opioids for the treatment of chronic pain and opioid- related addiction. The PCSS-B assists physicians in treating patients dependent on heroin or prescription opioid drugs with buprenorphine. Both provide training through webinars, online modules, peer support programs, listservs, virtual patients, and phone apps. HRSA plans to promote the availability of the PCSS-O and PCSS-B training to NHSC scholars and loan re- payers in field placement sites.

CIHS, ATTCs, and AHECs provide EBP training: Promotion of behavioral health EBP is provided regularly by the SAMHSA-HRSA CIHS, the SAMHSA ATTCs and the HRSA AHECs through webinars, conference training and dissemination of materials.

Technology in Training and Practice

Telebehavioral health activities: HRSA's BPHC and HAB collaborated with SAMHSA on the Secretary's Minority AIDS Initiative to expand HIV/AIDS care, viral hepatitis care, and behavioral health care to health centers through telehealth technology.

Medication Assisted Treatment (MAT) and telemedicine: SAMHSA has initiated a cross-agency discussion on the use of telemedicine to provide medication assisted treatment (MAT) to treat substance use disorders which will clarify current regulations around the prescription of controlled substances and the use of telemedicine. The goal is to establish clear standards and practice guidelines on the use of telemedicine in delivering MAT.

Other telehealth activities: HRSA's Office of Rural Health Policy (ORHP) and Office of Special Health Affairs (OSHA) are developing a telebehavioral services manual to encourage HRSA grantee providers to better incorporate the use of telehealth platforms for behavioral health services. In addition, ORHP's Office for the Advancement of Telehealth has numerous grants, some of which provide behavioral health services, promoting the use of telehealth technologies for health care delivery, education, and health information services.

Readiness of Safety Net Providers for Managed Care

Provider readiness: CIHS plans to host a webinar for behavioral health and primary care provider organizations on how to participate in managed behavioral health care provider networks. This web-based training will be held in collaboration with the Association for Behavioral Health and Wellness.

Non-Traditional Workforce

Paraprofessional training in SBIRT: SAMHSA's State SBIRT demonstration grants have focused on the training and utilization of paraprofessional staff including health educators, health navigators and health promotion advocates working under the supervision of licensed physicians or the health care system.

Report on bringing recovery services to scale: SAMHSA is preparing a report from an expert panel meeting on Peer Specialists and Recovery Coaches that was convened in March 2012 by Bringing Recovery Services to Scale – Technical Assistance Center Strategy (BRSS-TACS). It will include recommendations on increasing the utilization of peers in the behavioral health workforce.

Recovery to Practice: This SAMHSA effort is advancing a recovery-oriented approach to behavioral health care by developing, promoting, and disseminating training curricula on how to translate the concept of mental health recovery into practice.

Community Health Worker (CHW) curriculum and training: HRSA's AHEC program has implemented CHW training programs in collaboration with state and local partners, including the Department of Labor and Workforce Investment Boards. AHECs have trained CHWs on topics such as: cancer, diabetes, tobacco cessation and chronic disease self-management.

Promoting CHWs: Texas AHEC East worked with the Department of Labor to have CHWs deemed as an apprentice-able trade. Apprenticeship training is designed to prepare individuals for occupations and combines supervised on-the-job learning with classroom instruction.

APPENDIX B. REFERENCES

Anderson, C. (2012, March 12). Managing doctor, nurse practitioner turnover rates key to collaborative care|Healthcare Finance News. *Healthcare Finance News*. Retrieved from http://www.healthcarefinancenews.com/news/managing-doctor-nurse-practitioner- turnover-rates-key-delivery-collaborative-care-model.

Carise, D., Gurel, O., McMellan, A. T., Dugosh, K. & Kending, C. (2005). Getting patients the services they need using a computer-assisted system for patient assessment and referral referral? CASPAR. *Drug and Alcohol Dependence*, (80), 177-189. doi:10.1016/j.drugalcdep.2005.03.024.

Center for Substance Abuse Treatment. (2006). *Addiction Counseling Competencies: The Knowledge, Skills, and Attitudes of Professional Practice.* (Technical Assistance Publication Series 21. DHHS Publication No. SMA 08-4171). Rockville, MD: Substance Abuse and Mental Health Services Administration, (2006), reprinted 2007and 2008.

Center for Substance Abuse Treatment. (2007). *Competencies for Substance Abuse Treatment Clinical Supervisors.* (Technical Assistance Publication Series 21-A. DHHS Publication No. SMA 08-4243). Rockville, MD: Substance Abuse and Mental Health Services Administration reprinted 2008.

Center for Substance Abuse Treatment. (2009). *What Are Peer Recovery Support Services?* (HHS Publication No. SMA 09-4454.) Rockville, MD: Substance Abuse and Mental Health Services Administration.

Congressional Budget Office. (2012). *Estimates for the Insurance Coverage Provision of the Affordable Care Act Updated for the Recent Supreme Court Decision.* Retrieved January 4, 2013, from http://www.cbo.gov/publication/43472.

Congressional Budget Office. (2010). *Selected CBO publications related to health care legislation, (2009–2010).* Retrieved March 25, 2011, from http://www.cbo.gov/ftpdocs/120xx/doc12033/12-23-SelectedHealthcare Publications.pdf.

Curtis, S. L. & Eby, L. T. (2010). Recovery at work: The relationship between social identity and commitment among substance abuse counselors. *Journal of Substance Abuse Treatment, 39*, 248-254.

Daniels, A. S., Fricks, L. & Tunner, T. P., (Eds). (2011). *Pillars of Peer Support - Support -2: expanding the role of peer support services in mental health systems of care and recovery.* Retrieved February 2011, from http://www.pillarsofpeersupport.org/POPS2010-2.pdf.

Dilonardo, J. (2011). *Workforce Issues in Integrated Behavioral Healthcare: A Background Paper.* Unpublished Paper, National Council for Community Behavioral Healthcare.

Druss, B. G., Zhao, L., Von Esenwein, S., Morrato, E. H. & Marcus, S. C. (2011). Understanding excess mortality in persons with mental illness. *Medical Care, 49*(6), 599-604.

Delaney, K. R., Duffy, F. F., Dwyer, K. P., West, J. C., Wilk, J., Narrow, W. E., Hales, D. et al. (2002) Mental health practitioners and trainees. In Manderscheid, R.W., Henderson M.J., (Eds). *Mental Health, United State*

(327–368). Rockville, MD: Substance Abuse and Mental Health Services Administration.

Eby, L. T., Burke, H. & Maher, C. P. (2010). How serious of a problem is staff turnover in substance abuse treatment? A longitudinal study of actual turnover. *Journal of Substance Abuse Treatment, 39*, 264-271. doi:10.1016/j.jsat.2010.06.009.

Felitti, V. J., Anda, R. F., Nordenberg, D., Williamson, D. F., Spitz, A. M., Edwards, V. et al. (1998). Relationship of child abuse and household dysfunction to many of the leading causes of death in adults: The Adverse Childhood Experiences Study. *American Journal of Preventive Medicine, 14*, 245-258.

Friedli, L. & Parsonage, M. (2007). Mental health promotion: Building an economic case. *Northern Ireland Association for Mental Health.* Retrieved March 25, 2011, from http://www.chex.org.uk/uploads/ mhpeconomiccase.pdf?sess_scdc=ee4428ebde41914ab ac0e0535f55861c.

Garner, R., Hunter, B. D., Modisetter, K. C., Ihnes, P. C. & Godley, S. H. (2012). Treatment staff turnover in organizations implementing evidence-based practices: Turnover rates and their association with client outcomes. *Journal of Substance Abuse Treatment, 42*, 134-142.

Gaumond, P., Baytop, C. & Whitter, M. (2007). *Informing marketing strategies for recruitment into the addictions treatment workforce.* Abt Associates. Retrieved from http://partnersforrecovery.samhsa.gov/docs/ informing_marketing_strategies.pdf.

Gerson, L. W., Boex, J., Hua, K., Luckett, R. A., Zumbar, W. R., Bush, D. & Givens, C. (2001). Medical care used by treated and untreated substance abusing Medicaid patients. *Journal of Substance Abuse Treatment, 20*, 115-120.

Greiner, A. & Knebel, E. (Eds.). (2003). *Health professions education: A bridge to quality.* Washington, DC: National Academies Press.

Gulf Coast Addiction Technology Transfer Center. (2007). *Status of the workforce: addiction treatment in Texas - 2007 report.* ATTC Network. Retrieved from http://www.attcnetwork.org/userfiles/file/GulfCoast/ Texas_Addictions_Workforce_Rep ort_2007.pdf.

Institute of Medicine. (2006). *Improving the quality of health care for mental and substance-use conditions.* Washington, DC: National Academies Press.

Institute of Medicine. (2003). Greiner, A., & Knebel, E. (Eds.). *Health professions education: A bridge to quality.* Washington, DC: National Academies Press.

Institute of Medicine. (2004). Smedley, B. D., Butler, A. S., Bristow, L. R. (Eds.). *In the nation's compelling interest: Ensuring diversity in the health-care workforce.* Washington, DC: National Academies Press.

Institute of Medicine & Eden, J. (2012). *The mental health and substance use workforce for older adults: In whose hands?* Washington, DC: National Academies Press.

International Certification and Reciprocity Consortium. (2012, March 1) *Correspondence based on data from some member certification boards.*

Kaplan, L. (2003). *Substance abuse treatment workforce environmental scan.* (Contract No. 28298-006) Bethesda, MD: Abt Associates.

Knight, D. K., Becan, J. E. & Flynn, P. M. (2012). Organizational consequences of staff turnover in outpatient substance abuse treatment programs. *Journal of Substance Abuse Treatment, 42,* 143-150.

Knudsen, H. K., Ducharme, L. J. & Roman, P. (2008). Clinical supervision, emotional exhaustion, and turnover intention: A study of substance abuse treatment counselors in the Clinical Trials Network of the National Institute on Drug Abuse. *Journal of Substance Abuse Treatment, 35,* 387-395.

Knudsen, H. L., Ducharme, L. J. & Roman, P. (2006). Counselor emotional exhaustion and turnover intention in therapeutic communities. *Journal of Substance Abuse Treatment, 31,* 173-180.

Knudsen, H. K., Johnson, J.A. & Roman, P. M. (2003). Retaining counseling staff at substance abuse treatment centers: effects of management practices. *Journal of Substance Abuse Treatment, 24,* 129-135.

Knudsen, H. K., Oser, C. B., Abraham, A. J. & Roman, P. M. (2012). Physicians in the substance abuse treatment workforce: Understanding their employment within publicly funded treatment organizations. *Journal of Substance Abuse Treatment, 43,* 152-160.

Knudsen, J. R., Williams, A. M. & Perry, S. W. (2005). Tennessee Workforce Survey: Results of a Statewide Needs Assessment of Behavioral Health Professionals. *Central East Addiction Technology Transfer Center.* Retrieved from http://www.attcnetwork.org/explore/priorityareas/wfd/overview/documents/Central%20 East/TN_WorkforceReport_2004.pdf.

Leonardi, L. (2012). Five Low-Paying, High-Stress Jobs. *Career advice, interview questions, salary comparisons, and resume tips from Monster.* Retrieved from http://career- advice.monster.com/salary-benefits.

McLellan, A. T., Carise, D. & Kleber, H. D. (2003). Can the national addiction treatment infrastructure support the public's demand for quality care? *Journal of Substance Abuse Treatment, 25,* 117-121.

Mertens, J. R., Lu, Y. W., Parthasarathy, S., Moore, C. & Weisner, C. M. (2003). Medical and psychiatric conditions of alcohol and drug treatment patients in an HMO. *Archives of Internal Medicine, 163*, 2511-2517.

Mojtabai, R. & Olfson, M. (2011). Proportion of Antidepressants Prescribed Without A Psychiatric Diagnosis Is Growing. *Health Affairs, 30*(8), 1434-1442. doi:10.1377/hlthaff.2010.1024.

Mor Barak, M., Nissly, J. & Levin, A. (2001). Antecedents to retention and turnover among child welfare, social work, and other human service employees: What can we learn from past research? A review and metanalysis. *The Social Service Review, 75*(4), 625-667.

National Association of Alcoholism and Drug Abuse Counselors. (2003). *Practice Research Network. Report.* Author.

National Association of Community Health Centers. (2011). *NACHC 2010 Assessment of behavioral health services in federally qualified health centers.* Author. Retrieved from http://www.nachc.com/client/NACHC%202010%20Assessment%20of%20Behavioral%20Health%20Services%20in%20FQHCs_1_14_11_FINAL.pdf.

National Council for Community Behavioral Healthcare. (2011). *Behavioral health salary survey.* Retrieved from http://www.thenationalcouncil.org/cs/2011_behavioral_health_salary_survey.

New York State Office of Alcoholism and Substance Abuse Services. (2002). *The addictions profession: a workforce in crisis. A compilation of the results of the 2001 regional workforce development focus groups.* Author.

Parks, J. & National Association of State Mental Health Program Directors. (2006). *Morbidity and mortality in people with serious mental illness.* Alexandria, VA: National Association of State Mental Health Program Directors Medical Directors Council.

Plomondon, M. E., Magid, D. J., Steiner, J. F., MaWhinney, S., Gifford, B. D., Shih, S. C., Grunwald, G. K. et al. (2007). Primary care provider turnover and quality in managed care organizations. *American Journal of Managed Care, 13*(8), 465-472.

RMC Research Corporation. (2003). *Advancing the current state of addiction treatment. A regional needs assessment of substance abuse treatment professionals in the pacific northwest.* Portland, OR. Author.

RMC Research Corporation. (2003a). *Kentucky workforce survey 2002. Results of a statewide needs assessment of substance abuse treatment professionals.* Portland, OR: Author.

Ryan, O., Murphy, D. & Krom, L. (2012). *Vital Signs: Taking the Pulse of the Addiction Treatment Workforce, A National Report - Executive Summary.*

Kansas City, MO: Addiction Technology Transfer Center National Office in residence at the University of Missouri-Kansas City.

Salzer, M. S., Schwenk, E. S. & Brsilovskiy, E. (2010). Certified Peer Specialist Roles and Activities: Results from a National Survey. *Psychiatric Services, 61*(5), 520-523.

Substance Abuse and Mental Health Services Administration. (2006). *Report to Congress Addiction Treatment Workforce Development.* Retrieved from http://partnersforrecovery.samhsa.gov/docs/Report_to_Congress.pdf.

Substance Abuse and Mental Health Services Administration. (2006a). *Strengthening Professional Identity: Challenges of the Addiction Treatment Workforce.* Retrieved from http://partnersforrecovery.samhsa.gov/docs/Strengthening_Professional_Identity.pdf.

Substance Abuse and Mental Health Services Administration. (2007). *An Action Plan for Behavioral Health Workforce Development.* (HHS Publication No. SMA 11-4629.) Rockville, MD: Substance Abuse and Mental Health Services Administration. Retrieved from: http://www.samhsa.gov/workforce/annapolis/workforceactionplan.pdf.

Substance Abuse and Mental Health Services Administration. (2008). *Unpublished. SAMHSA data, 2008 National Survey of Mental Health Treatment Facilities.*

Substance Abuse and Mental Health Services Administration. (2009). *What are Peer Recovery Support Services?* Retrieved from http://store.samhsa.gov/shin/content//SMA09- 4454/SMA09-4454.pdf.

Substance Abuse and Mental Health Services Administration. (2010). *Mental Health, United States, 2008.* (HHS Publication No. SMA 10-4590.) Rockville, MD: Substance Abuse and Mental Health Services Administration.

Substance Abuse and Mental Health Services Administration. (2010). *National survey of substance abuse treatment services: Data on substance abuse treatment facilities.* Rockville, MD: Substance Abuse and Mental Health Services Administration.

Substance Abuse and Mental Health Services Administration. (2011a). *Leading Change: A Plan for SAMHSA's Roles and Actions 2011-2014.* (HHS Publication No. SMA 11-4629). Rockville, MD: Substance Abuse and Mental Health Services Administration.

Substance Abuse and Mental Health Services Administration. (2011b). *Scopes of Practice and Career Ladder for Substance Use Disorders Counseling.* http://store.samhsa.gov/product/Scopes-of-Practice-and-Career-Ladder-for-Substance- Use-Disorders-Counseling/PEP11-SCOPES.

Substance Abuse and Mental Health Services Administration. (2011). *Results from the 2010 National Survey on Drug Use and Health: Summary of national findings*. (NSDUH Series H-41, HHS Publication No. (SMA) 11-4658). Rockville, MD: Substance Abuse and Mental Health Services Administration.

Substance Abuse and Mental Health Services Administration (2012a). *Mental Health, United States, 2010*. (HHS Publication No. (SMA) 12-4681). Rockville, MD: Substance Abuse and Mental Health Services Administration, Center for Mental Health Services.

Substance Abuse and Mental Health Services Administration. (2012b). *Results from the 2011 National Survey on Drug Use and Health: Summary of national findings*. Rockville, MD: Substance Abuse and Mental Health Services Administration, Center for Behavioral Health Statistics and Quality.

Substance Abuse and Mental Health Services Administration. (2012). *Treatment Episode Data Set: 2001-2010. National Admissions to Substance Abuse Treatment Services*. (DASIS Series S-61, Publication No. SMA 12-4701.) Rockville, MD: Substance Abuse and Mental Health Services Administration, Center for Behavioral Health Statistics and Quality.

Substance Abuse and Mental Health Services Administration & National Association of State Mental Health Program Directors. (2004). *The damaging consequences of violence and trauma*. Retrieved from http://www.nasmhpd.org/general_files/publications/ntac.

Thomas, M., (February, 2006). State Medicaid Strategies for Integrated Care: Health Plan Experience, a Presentation to RWJ Depression in Primary Care Annual Meeting.

Thomas, K. C., Ellis, A. R., Konard, T. R., Holzer, C. E. & Morrissey, J. P. (2009). County- level Estimates of Mental Health Professional Shortage in the United States. *Psychiatric Services*, *60*(10), 1323-1328.

Touhy, C. M. (2006). Blueprint for the States: Policies to Improve the Way States Organize and Deliver Alcohol and Drug Prevention Treatment. *National Association for Alcoholism and Drug Abuse Counselors*. Retrieved from http://www.naadac.org/component/content/article/54-resources/349-pr175.

U.S. Census Bureau (2010). 2010 Census. *Census Bureau*. Retrieved from http://www.census.gov/2010census/

Unützer, J., Katon, W. J., Fan, M. Y., Schoenbaum, M. C., Lin, E. H., Della Penna, R. D. & Powers, D. (2008). Long-term cost effects of collaborative care for late-life depression. *American Journal of Managed Care, 14*(2), 95-100.

Woltmann, E. M., Whitley, R., McHugo, G. J., Brunette, M., Torrey, W. C., Coots, L., Lynde, D. et al. (2008). The Role of Staff Turnover in the Implementation of Evidence-Based Practices in Mental Health Care. *Psychiatric Services, 59*(7), 732-737. doi:10.1176/appi.ps.59.7.732.

End Notes

[1] In this report, the term "behavioral health" is used to encompass mental health conditions, mental illness, substance abuse, substance use disorders, and addictions. In various contexts, the term is used to include emotional health development, substance abuse and mental illness prevention services and activities, treatment services, and/or recovery support activities and services for those in recovery from mental illness, mental health problems, and/or addictions.

[2] There are credentialing boards for addiction counselors in all 50 States; however, not all of them collect data on a consistent basis nor do they all collect data on the same variables. Therefore in several places in this Demographic Information section the numbers of certification boards responding may vary.

[3] The Mental Health HPSAs do not include consideration of shortages of specialty addiction services professionals.

[4] All salary data are provided by online salary database PayScale.com. Salaries listed are median, annual salaries for full-time workers with five to eight years of experience and include all bonuses, commissions or profit-sharing.

[5] A summary of current HRSA and SAMHSA workforce activities related to topics raised or addressed at the joint listening session are captured in Appendix A, some of which are also captured in the body of this report.

In: America's Substance Abuse ...
Editor: Omri Galinsky

ISBN: 978-1-62808-634-8
© 2013 Nova Science Publishers, Inc.

Chapter 2

REPORT TO CONGRESS: ADDICTIONS TREATMENT WORKFORCE DEVELOPMENT[*]

Substance Abuse and Mental Health Services Administration

EXECUTIVE SUMMARY

In 2004, over 23 million Americans age 12 and older needed specialty treatment for alcohol or illicit drug problems (NSDUH, 2005). The human, social and economic costs of not treating substance use disorders are indisputable. Yet, substance use disorders treatment systems are constrained by an inadequate infrastructure to support current and future demands for treatment. The addictions treatment field is facing a workforce crisis. Worker shortages, inadequate compensation, insufficient professional development and stigma currently challenge the field. Increasingly, treatment and recovery support providers also struggle with issues related to recruitment, retention and professional development of staff. The ability to provide quality addictions treatment and recovery support services is severely hampered by these conditions.

---

[*] This is an edited, reformatted and augmented version of the Substance Abuse and Mental Health Services Administration, dated 2006.

In its report on the Fiscal Year (FY) 2006 budget for the Department of Health and Human Services (DHHS), the House Committee on Appropriations stated the following:

> The Committee has concerns that people who are seeking substance abuse treatment are unable to access services due to the lack of an adequate clinical treatment workforce. People seeking treatment often have to wait for weeks or months before they are accepted into a treatment facility. The Committee requests that SAMHSA issue a report, after consultation with stakeholders and other Federal partners, on workforce development for substance abuse treatment professionals. The report should focus on both the recruitment and retention of counselors and on improving the skills of those already providing services as well as ways in which States can play a role. The Committee requests that this report be transmitted to the House and Senate Committees on Appropriations by March 1, 2006. (House report No. 109-143, page 117)

This report was prepared in response to the Committee request. It summarizes trends in addictions treatment and the challenges that confront the treatment workforce. Importantly, it also articulates the perspectives of stakeholders and Federal partners by presenting a series of recommendations aimed at strengthening the field's professional identity. The recommendations in this report reflect some of the best thinking in the field and are intended to provide momentum for ongoing discussions among stakeholders about specific implementation strategies. The report discusses current trends in funding, staff recruitment and retention, patient characteristics and clinical practice and identifies recommendations in the following six areas: infrastructure; leadership and management; recruitment; education and accreditation; retention; and priorities for further study. This report focuses on all professionals who provide addictions treatment and recovery support services, e.g., addictions counselors, physicians, psychologists, nurses, outreach and intake workers, case managers, social workers, marriage and family therapists, recovery support workers and clergy.

BACKGROUND AND APPROACH

Workforce development has been a principal area of concern for SAMHSA for many years. In recognition of the mounting workforce crisis, SAMHSA recently elevated workforce development to a program priority on its "SAMHSA Priorities: Programs and Principles Matrix." This designation will result in greater attention to this critical issue. This report was based, in part, on an environmental scan of recent research related to the treatment workforce.

SAMHSA subsequently convened 128 individuals representing diverse stakeholder groups in nine separate stakeholder meetings. During these meetings, SAMHSA solicited information and recommendations from representatives knowledgeable about the exceptional challenges faced by the addictions treatment workforce. The environmental scan provided a starting point for stakeholder discussions. Individuals from the following organizations and employment categories provided input: addictions counselors, Addiction Technology Transfer Centers (ATTCs), certification boards, Federal agencies, professional trade associations, clinical supervisors, college and university professors, faith-based providers, human resource managers, marriage and family therapists, nurses, physicians, psychiatrists, recovery support personnel, researchers, social workers, and State Directors. The participating Federal government partners represented a wide range of agencies, including the Departments of Labor, Defense (Marine Corps and Navy), Veterans Affairs, Justice and Education, as well as the National Institute on Drug Abuse, the National Institute on Alcohol Abuse and Alcoholism, the Health Resources and Services Administration, the Centers for Medicare and Medicaid Services, and each of the SAMHSA Centers.

CONTEXT: TRENDS IMPACTING THE WORKFORCE

This report begins with a discussion of both long-term and emergent issues impacting the addictions treatment workforce. The information included in this section provides a context for understanding the challenges facing the addictions treatment workforce and a background for the recommendations that follow.

Among the key issues facing the workforce are:

- Insufficient workforce/treatment capacity to meet demand;
- The changing profile of those needing services (e.g., an increasing number of injecting drug users, narcotic prescription and methamphetamine users);
- A shift to increased public financing of treatment;
- Challenges related to the adoption of best practices;

- Increased utilization of medications in treatment;
- A movement toward a recovery management model of care (i.e., a chronic care approach analogous to those adopted for the treatment of other chronic disorders, such as diabetes and heart disease);
- Provision of services in generalist and specialist settings (e.g., provision of services in primary care and other settings in addition to addictions treatment program settings);
- Use of performance and patient outcome measures; and
- Discrimination associated with addictions.

STAKEHOLDER PRIORITY RECOMMENDATIONS BY FOCUS AREA

Following the context discussion, the report includes a listing of stakeholder priority recommendations for key focus areas and a detailed discussion for each focus area and recommendation. In total, 20 stakeholder recommendations are presented in this report.

A. Infrastructure Development Priorities

1. Create career paths for the treatment and recovery workforce and adopt national core competency standards;
2. Foster network development; and
3. Provide technical assistance to enhance the capacity to use information technology.

B. Leadership and Management Priorities

1. Develop, deliver and sustain training for treatment and recovery support supervisors, who serve as the technology transfer agents for the latest research and best practices; and
2. Develop, deliver and sustain leadership and management development initiatives.

C. Recruitment Priorities

1. Expand recruitment of health care professionals in addictions medicine;
2. Improve student recruitment with educational institutions, focusing on under-represented groups;
3. Employ marketing strategies to attract workers to the addictions treatment field; and
4. Continue efforts to reduce the stigma associated with working in addictions treatment.

D. Addictions Education and Accreditation Priorities

1. Include training on addictions as part of education programs for primary health care and for other health and human service professions (e.g., physicians, nurses, psychologists and social workers);
2. Call for the use of national addictions core competencies as the basis of curricula;
3. Support the development and adoption of national accreditation standards for addictions education programs;
4. Encourage national and State boards for the health professions to have at least 10 percent of licensing examination questions pertain to addictions;
5. Support academic programs in Historically Black Colleges and Universities (HBCUs), Hispanic Serving Institutions, Tribal Colleges and Universities and other minority- serving institutions; and
6. Develop college and university courses on health services research and its application; and systematically disseminate research findings to academic institutions.

E. Retention Priorities

1. Identify and disseminate best practices in staff retention; and
2. Address substance misuse and relapse within the workforce.

F. Study Priorities

1. Conduct studies that examine the relationships among level of education, type of education, training and treatment outcomes;
2. Conduct studies that examine the relationships among clinician and patient/client cultural, demographic and other characteristics, therapeutic alliance and treatment outcomes; and
3. Conduct studies that explore questions related to the characteristics of clinicians' training and skills that enhance therapeutic alliance.

NEXT STEPS

This report, developed by SAMHSA with the guidance of expert stakeholders from the addictions treatment and recovery field and representatives of other Federal agencies, identifies and discusses current and emerging issues in the area of workforce development in the addictions treatment field. The future effectiveness of the addictions treatment workforce rests on its ability to develop systems to address issues of recruitment, retention, and staff development. Other health care professions (e.g. nurses and physicians) have demonstrated that such efforts can prove effective. It is time that the addictions treatment field in partnership with States and the Federal government follow that example, taking the steps necessary to address the challenges faced by the addictions treatment workforce.

INTRODUCTION

A Workforce in Crisis: New Opportunities for Change

Addictions treatment is facing a workforce crisis. High turnover rates, worker shortages, an aging workforce, inadequate compensation, insufficient professional development, lack of defined career paths and stigma currently challenge the field. These deficiencies have a direct impact on workers and the patients/clients under their care. Further challenging the workforce are an increasingly complex patient/client population, the demand for greater accountability in patient care, limited access to information technology and the need to rapidly incorporate scientific advances into the treatment process. The addictions treatment field is composed of workers from many different professions (e.g., counselors, physicians, nurses, social workers, psychologists, marriage and family therapists, outreach and intake workers, case managers and clergy). This diversity gives the field a rich array of perspectives and skills, but also requires complex, coordinated responses to workforce issues. While the majority of practitioners in the addictions treatment field are counselors, the roles of all professions involved in the provision of addictions treatment are critically important.

Even as the treatment system struggles with these challenges, the foundation is solidly in place to strengthen the professional identity of the workforce. The progress in science and the emerging consensus about the need for academic accreditation and national core competencies provide opportunities for the workforce to move forward with new resolve. The field is at a pivotal point in the development of its workforce. By investing in the chief asset of the treatment system—the individuals who provide addictions treatment and recovery services—significant progress can be made to address critical workforce issues.

Workforce issues in health care have gained recent prominence on the national agenda. In 2001, for example, the Institute of Medicine (IOM) produced a landmark report, *Crossing the Quality Chasm: A New Health System for the 21st Century*, which concluded that the U.S. health care system needs fundamental change. Report recommendations included a framework and strategies for achieving substantial improvements, including six approaches to improve health care and ten rules to guide the redesign of the health care system. In 2005, the IOM report *Improving the Quality of Health Care for Mental and Substance-Use Conditions* included a dedicated chapter discussing the need to increase substance use and mental health workforce capacity for quality improvement. While SAMHSA has been addressing workforce issues for more than a decade, these issues have been further elevated due to concerns regarding recruitment, staff retention, and adoption of best practices raised by the diverse professions that comprise the workforce.

In 1999, prior to the IOM report, SAMHSA convened a Workforce Issues Panel as part of the National Treatment Plan initiative to examine workforce issues related to addictions treatment. The Panel recommended (1) creating a national platform within SAMHSA to address addictions workforce issues; (2) developing and strengthening an infrastructure to attract, support and maintain a competent and diverse workforce representative of the patient/client population; and improving workforce competency by providing education and training rooted in evidence- based knowledge.

Recognizing the need for more comprehensive information about the workforce, SAMHSA commissioned an environmental scan of recent research related to the treatment workforce. The environmental scan identified five specific needs:

- Quantitative data on the workforce;
- Educational standards and workforce credentialing;
- Training to raise skill levels of the existing workforce;
- Strategies to reduce stigma; and
- Strategies to address an aging workforce (Kaplan, 2003).

Using the environmental scan as a starting point for discussions, SAMHSA convened 128 individuals representing diverse stakeholder groups in nine separate meetings. During these meetings, SAMHSA solicited information and recommendations from representatives knowledgeable about the exceptional challenges faced by the addictions treatment workforce. Individuals from the following organizations and employment categories provided input: addictions counselors, ATTCs, certification boards, Federal agencies, professional trade associations, clinical supervisors, college and university professors, faith-based providers, human resource managers, marriage and family therapists, nurses, physicians, psychiatrists, recovery support personnel, researchers, social workers, State Directors and treatment providers. This report includes recommendations that emerged from these expert panels.

Congress, concerned that individuals cannot access treatment because of a clinical workforce shortage, called on SAMHSA, as the lead substance abuse services agency, to develop a workforce development report for substance abuse treatment professionals. H. Rpt.109-143 required that the report be developed in consultation with stakeholders and Federal partners and focus on both the recruitment and retention of counselors and on improving the skills of those already providing services. It also required that the report identify ways in which States can address the workforce crisis.

The Evolution of the Addictions Treatment Workforce

The addictions treatment workforce is composed of highly committed practitioners, in a number of different professions, who care for patients/clients with substance use disorders. Each of these groups contributes to a comprehensive treatment and recovery process. Recovering individuals have been a critically important component of the workforce from the inception of the field. They serve as trained professionals, as specialized recovery support workers and as volunteers. The nature of the addictions treatment workforce has changed substantially over the past 40 years. Prior to the mid-1970s, recovering individuals provided counseling services with minimal formal training. In the late 1970s, States and national associations established professional standards and credentialing processes (Keller and Dermatis, 1999). Credentialing bodies now exist in every State, and a college degree is the norm rather than the exception for professionals in the field. Eighty percent of direct care treatment staff, for example, hold a bachelor's degree (Johnson et al., 2002; Knudsen et al., 2003; RMC Research Corporation, 2003) and 53 percent have a master's degree or above (Harwood, 2002).

Remarkable advances in scientific knowledge, professional development and standards of care have enabled addictions treatment to emerge as a specialty health care discipline. However, problems related to infrastructure, recruitment, retention and education, and training of the workforce create an environment in which it is increasingly difficult to implement the most effective treatment. The challenges to maintaining a qualified workforce are numerous. Greater academic demands are being placed on treatment professionals. Many individuals who have traditionally entered the workforce may be discouraged from working in the field, either because of the increasing academic requirements, because compensation is inadequate to justify the investment of time and monetary resources required to obtain additional educational training, or because workloads and schedules make it difficult or impossible to complete the required academic training.

As scientific knowledge in the field of addictions treatment has expanded and the levels of credentialing have increased, one thing has remained constant: the exceptional level of passion and dedication that counselors, other professionals in the field and volunteers bring to their work. While the field currently faces a variety of challenges, the sense of mission that drives the treatment workforce gives it both a unique history and a unique resilience. Efforts to address workforce issues in the addictions treatment field need to build on this foundation and tap into the extraordinary assets that addictions treatment professionals regularly evidence.

Organization of This Report

This report consists of four sections:

- Section I: Context: Trends Impacting the Workforce
- Section II: Stakeholder Recommendations
  A. Infrastructure Development Priorities
  B. Leadership and Management Priorities
  C. Recruitment Priorities
  D. Addictions Education and Accreditation Priorities
  E. Retention Priorities
  F. Study Priorities
- Section III: Conclusion
- Section IV: References

Section I provides a historical context, demographics, and regulatory and practice trends relevant to understanding current workforce issues and the kinds of strategies that will be required to address them. This section provides a background for the recommendations that follow. Section II presents recommendations that emerged from the SAMHSA-sponsored stakeholder meetings. Although these categories overlap, they provide a useful framework for a systematic analysis of the recommendations. Section III concludes the report. Section IV contains the references included in the report.

I. CONTEXT: TRENDS IMPACTING THE WORKFORCE

The purpose of this section is to provide a context for understanding and addressing both long- standing and emergent workforce issues. The addictions treatment field and the social, economic and political contexts in which the workforce operates have evolved significantly over the past 30 years. While many of the challenges facing the addictions treatment workforce have remained relatively constant over time, others have emerged more recently.

Among the key issues facing the workforce are:

- Insufficient workforce/treatment capacity to meet demand;
- The changing profile of those needing services;
- A shift to increased public financing of treatment;

Report to Congress: Addictions Treatment Workforce Development   89

- Challenges related to the adoption of best practices;
- Increased utilization of medications in treatment;
- A movement toward a recovery management model of care;
- Provision of services in generalist and specialist settings;
- Use of performance and patient outcome measures; and
- Discrimination associated with addictions.

Each of these issues is discussed below.

Insufficient Workforce to Meet Treatment Demands

Nationally, addictions treatment capacity is insufficient to accommodate all those seeking services and is substantially inadequate to serve the total population in need. Capacity issues vary by geographic area, population and the type of treatment required. Per capita funding for treatment services also differs by State. Some States are able to invest substantial State and local resources into treatment, whereas others rely primarily on Federal funding. Given limited resources, States and localities are faced with difficult decisions, such as limiting the types or number of services individuals can receive and/or limiting the number of individuals who can receive services. Moreover, in recent years, many States have experienced severe revenue shortfalls that have reduced treatment capacity, despite Federal budget increases.

When treatment systems are required to provide additional services with less funding, providers and the workforce experience enormous pressures. Additionally, a large number of individuals are unable to access care due to limited workforce capacity.

The *2004 National Survey on Drug Use and Health* (NSDUH, 2005), which collected data on self-reported drug and alcohol use, found that:

- Approximately 23.48 million individuals age 12 and older needed specialty treatment for alcohol or illicit drug problems;
- 2.33 million of these individuals received treatment at a specialty facility;
- Of the 21.15 million persons who were determined to need but did not receive treatment, only 1.2 million acknowledged a need for treatment; and

- Of the 1.2 million persons who felt that they needed treatment, 792,000 did not attempt to access it, and 441,000 reported that they were unable to access treatment.

The high costs of not treating alcohol and drug abuse are well documented. Economic costs associated with alcohol abuse are estimated to be $184.6 billion and the costs of drug abuse are estimated to be $143 billion (Mark et al., 2005). These include the medical costs associated with alcohol and drug abuse, lost earnings linked to premature death, lost productivity, motor vehicle crashes, crime and other social consequences. The data further reflect that treating substance use disorders can result in cost benefits for many other systems, such as primary health care, child welfare, welfare and criminal justice (NIDA, 1999).

The capacity constraints that the field faces go beyond limited treatment resources. Capacity is also limited by the lack of a sufficient number of skilled practitioners. Treatment capacity at any level cannot exist without a viable workforce, and treatment organizations are currently struggling to recruit, hire, train and retain staff to respond to the demand for services. When available, increases in treatment dollars are primarily used to expand capacity to serve the greatest number of individuals, often neglecting the workforce infrastructure. Low salaries, minimal benefits, high turnover and staff dissatisfaction make recruiting staff to expand capacity a mounting challenge. (A table showing the median salary of addictions counselors and of similar professions in 2000, the most recent year for which data is available, can be found in Section II, under *Retention Issues*, below.) Additionally, the emergent issues discussed in this section are creating further pressure on an inadequately sized workforce that is battling to keep pace with these new demands. To meet these demands, the workforce will need to adopt a new way of doing business. Intensive technology transfer efforts will be required to make this possible.

The Changing Profile of Those Needing Services

Over the past decade, drug use patterns and resultant treatment needs have substantively changed.

- The preferred route of drug administration among youth changed from inhalation to injection from 1992 to 2000, with the rate of injection among heroin users increasing from 34 to 51 percent among those

under age 18 and from 48 to 63 percent among those ages 18 to 24 (SAMHSA, 2003).
- The numbers of persons using prescription pain relievers non-medically for the first time increased from 600,000 in 1990 to more than 2 million in 2001 (NSDUH, 2004a).
- The number of older adults with substance use disorders is expected to increase from 2.5 million persons in 1999 to 5 million persons by 2020, a 100 percent increase (Gfroerer et al., 2002).

Admission patterns to treatment facilities also changed significantly from 1992 to 2002 (see Figure 1 below). For instance, admissions for alcohol dependence and abuse declined from 59 percent to 42 percent, and admissions for cocaine declined from 18 percent to 13 percent. These decreases were offset, however, by increases in admissions for marijuana/hashish users from 6 percent to 15 percent, for primary opiate users from 12 percent to 18 percent and for stimulant users from 1 percent to 7 percent. Among youth 15 to 17 years of age, admissions for marijuana rose from 23 percent to 63 percent (SAMHSA, 2004b). These data point to the necessity of having a workforce prepared to respond to changes in both drug use and patient characteristics.

The complex constellation of conditions with which individuals often present to treatment, including co-occurring mental health and substance use disorders, co-morbid medical conditions, homelessness and criminal justice or child welfare system involvement, places exceptional demands on the workforce and requires a sophisticated, multi-disciplinary approach that bridges the mental health, medical and other systems.

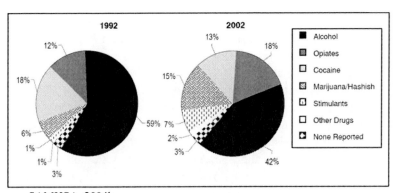

Source: SAMHSA, 2004b.

Figure 1. Primary Substance at Admission: 1992 and 2002.

Practitioners in generalist settings are beginning to screen for hazardous substance use patterns and potential addictive disorders. Such screening now occurs in hospitals, emergency rooms, ambulatory clinics and other medical and non-medical settings. This practice will likely result in individuals presenting for specialty addictions services earlier in the progression of their addictive disorders. As protocols for Screening, Brief Intervention and Referral to Treatment (SBIRT) are adopted more broadly, the professionals in the addictions treatment field will increasingly be faced with two populations that, heretofore, have typically not been served. These are (1) individuals who are just beginning the progression to dependence; and (2) individuals with diagnosable dependence disorders, who are not yet ready to initiate traditional treatment but who may be willing to engage in low-demand motivational interventions that could eventually lead to treatment. Staff will need to be trained to effectively engage patients/clients in a manner that is fully cognizant of and responsive to both their clinical presentation and their readiness for change.

For many organizations, it will be a significant challenge to develop the capacity to more effectively treat those who are multiply impaired, those who are just beginning the progression toward dependence and those who, while dependent, are not yet ready to engage in treatment. Growing evidence indicates that the addictions treatment field must be prepared to serve populations that present with increasing levels of impairment across multiple domains, as well as populations that present earlier in the progression of a substance use disorder than in the past. Four trends related to increased severity cause concern.

- **Increased potency of illegal drugs such as marijuana and heroin.** The University of Mississippi's 2000 Marijuana Potency Monitoring Project showed that commercial grade marijuana tetrahydrocannabinol (THC) levels rose from under 2 percent in the late 1970s and early 1980s to 6.1 percent in 2000 (DEA, 2003). Also, data from the System to Retrieve Information from Drug Evidence (STRIDE) showed that the nationwide average purity for heroin from all sources measured approximately 37 percent in 2000, in contrast to 26 percent in 1991 and 7 percent in 1980 (DEA, 2001).
- **Consumption of dangerous and illegal drugs among younger users and, in particular, increased heroin addictions within this population.** The availability of high-purity heroin, which can be

snorted, has given rise to a new generation of younger users (DEA, 2001).

- **Serious medical problems among the patient/client population.** Increasingly, addictions programs are treating patients/clients with serious medical problems. According to the Centers for Disease Control and Prevention (CDC), the number of individuals living with AIDS who were exposed by injection drug use increased from 55,735 in 1998 to 68,636 in 2002, an increase of 23.1 percent (CDC, 2002a). Viral hepatitis is also a significant problem among injection drug users (IDUs). According to the CDC, 17,000 (60 percent) of the 30,000 new cases of hepatitis C in 2000 occurred among IDUs. Hepatitis B and C infections are also acquired rapidly among IDUs. Within five years of beginning drug use, 50 to 70 percent of IDUs contract hepatitis B, while 50 to 80 percent contract hepatitis C (CDC, 2002b).

  The rapid growth in methamphetamine use has led to a range of serious health problems among users. Cardiovascular problems associated with methamphetamine use include rapid heart rate, irregular heartbeat, increased blood pressure and damage to small blood vessels in the brain that can lead to stroke. Acute lead poisoning is also a growing problem among methamphetamine users, since a common method of illegal production uses lead acetate as a reagent (NIDA, 2002). Because lead poisoning in adults is associated with increased incidence of depression, aggressive behavior, antisocial behavior and brain damage, the treatment of patients/clients with lead exposure is challenging (NIDA, 2002).

- **Complex co-occurring disorders.** Complex co-occurring disorders are a significant issue among individuals in addictions treatment. According to the National Survey on Drug Use and Health (NSDUH), there were an estimated 21.4 million adults aged 18 or older with Serious Psychological Distress (SPD) in 2004. This represents 9.9 percent of all adults compared to the rate of 8.3 percent found in 2002. Among adults with SPD in 2004, 21.3 percent were dependent on or abused alcohol or illicit drugs compared to 7.9 percent of adults not experiencing SPD (SAMHSA, 2005). An even larger concern is the number of individuals entering addictions treatment with a mild or moderate mental illness.

  With respect to these individuals, the *2001-2002 National Epidemiologic Survey on Alcohol and Related Conditions* (NESARC) found that 19.7 percent of the respondents with any substance use disorder had at least one independent mood disorder during the same 12-month period. Furthermore, 17.7 percent had at least one independent anxiety disorder. Of those who sought treatment for an alcohol use disorder, 40.7 percent had at least one independent mood disorder, 33.4 percent had an independent anxiety disorder, and 33.0 percent had a drug use disorder. Moreover, among respondents with any drug use disorder who sought treatment for that disorder, 60.0 percent had at least one independent mood disorder, 42.6 percent had at least one independent anxiety disorder and 55.7 percent had a co-morbid alcohol use disorder (Grant et al., 2004). Only 9.9 percent of individuals who needed specialty addictions treatment in 2004 accessed care (NSDUH, 2005).

The NESARC provides evidence that mood and anxiety disorders must be addressed in the specialty addictions setting and that alcohol and drug use disorders must be dealt with in the generalist and specialty mental health settings. The study authors emphasize the seriousness of both substance induced and independent mood and anxiety disorders. "Substance induced disorders," the authors point out, "have been shown to increase the risk for poor outcome of substance dependence and lifetime number of suicide attempts." Untreated, independent mood and anxiety disorders among individuals receiving addictions treatment can lead not only to relapse, but also to suicide. "Short of this ultimately adverse outcome, independent mood and anxiety disorders, particularly among individuals who have a co-morbid substance use disorder, are immensely disabling" (Grant et al., 2004).

Shift to Increased Public Financing of Treatment

Individuals with substance use disorders rely on public sources of funding to a much greater extent than people with other diseases. According to *National Expenditures for Mental Health Services and Substance Abuse Treatment 1991-2001*, 76 percent of total substance use spending was from public sources, while only 45 percent of all health care was publicly financed (Mark et al., 2005). During the 10-year period covered by the report, public expenditures for substance use grew by 6.8 percent annually whereas overall public health care expenditures grew by 7.2 percent annually. Notably, private payer expenditures in the form of insurance reimbursements for substance abuse services trended in the opposite direction, falling by 1.1 percent annually while overall insurance expenditures for health care increased by 6.9 percent annually during that period. Out-of-pocket spending for addictions-related services grew by 3.2 percent annually, compared to 3.8 percent for all health (Mark et al., 2005). (See Figure 2 below.)

This study points to the fact that the majority of substance use disorder treatment is financed by the public sector, that this trend is continuing and that care for substance use disorders is not financed in the same manner as other health care conditions. Though addictions impact all segments of society, lack of health coverage for treatment places enormous demands on the publicly funded system and its workforce. Given current pressures on public funding of treatment services, particularly at the State and local levels, this decline in private insurance coverage is especially onerous.

Challenges Related to the Adoption of Best Practices

The adoption of best practices requires a stable infrastructure, organizational commitment and staff development. Indeed, the gap between what we know and what we practice is sizeable. Increasingly, the workforce is assimilating best practices into its work. Practitioners are replacing unproven approaches, involving confrontation, with research-based approaches such as brief intervention, brief treatment, motivational interviewing and motivational enhancement techniques, social skills training, contingency management and community reinforcement. Many of these clinical approaches primarily focus on the use of objective feedback and empathic listening to increase a person's awareness of the potential problems caused, consequences experienced and the risks faced as a result of substance use (Rollnick and Miller, 1995).

Although the field has progressed toward incorporating best practices into its work, significant disparity remains between approaches indicated by research findings and those typically implemented by programs. Hennessy reports that the average time lag between development of an innovative practice and its adoption in practice is 17 years (Hennessy, 2004). Barriers that impede the use of evidence-based health services include resistance to change by entrenched and threatened organizational structures, outdated reimbursement rules, lack of effective provider training and lack of resources (Corrigan et al., 2001). Given these challenges related to transferring new knowledge into practice, individuals who access addictions treatment will often not receive the interventions that current research indicates are the most likely to assist them in achieving positive outcomes.

Increased Utilization of Medications in Treatment

Since the 1980s, medications for treating substance use disorders have become more available. Advances in this area have implications for improving treatment outcomes and the quality of life for patients/clients. Combining pharmacological and behavioral treatments often improves patient/client response better than either component alone. For example, just as high cholesterol can be dramatically reduced by combining diet and exercise with cholesterol-lowering medications, risk of relapse for an alcohol-dependent person can be reduced by administration of naltrexone in combination with treatment and community-based supports. Addictive disorders mirror other chronic disorders in that they often respond better to treatment approaches that extend over time, addressing physiological and neurological components of the disorder in addition to providing strategies and supports to replace unhealthy patterns with healthy ones.

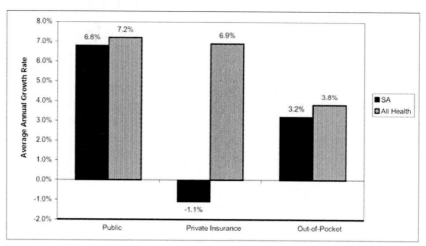

Source: Mark et al., 2005.

Figure 2. Growth of Public, Private Insurance and Out-of-Pocket Payments for Substance Abuse (SA) versus All Health, 1991-2001.

Medications are used for detoxification, co-morbid psychiatric conditions, opioid agonist/antagonist therapy, office-based opioid treatment, maintenance of abstinence and pain management. For example, the approval of buprenorphine by the Food and Drug Administration (FDA) provides a viable option (in addition to methadone) for addressing opiate addictions. Because it has been approved as an office-based opioid addiction treatment, buprenorphine has the potential to expand access to services by making them available in settings previously not possible, i.e., physician practices. In addition, disulfiram (antabuse) has long been used to assist individuals with alcohol dependence to abstain. Naltrexone has also been used to assist alcoholics and opiate addicts in maintaining abstinence. In July 2004, the FDA approved campral ® (acamprosate) for assisting individuals in maintaining abstinence after withdrawing from alcohol. Acamprosate is the first medication approved for the treatment of alcoholism in a decade.

The prevalence of co-occurring mental health disorders generally requires concurrent pharmacological and psychosocial interventions, making psychotropic medications an increasingly significant component of the addictions treatment process. Moreover, the high rates of co-morbid chronic medical disorders and contagious conditions with which individuals seeking publicly funded treatment present require that programs have the ability to administer and monitor a broad array of medications, to treat conditions ranging from hypertension and high serum cholesterol to tuberculosis, hepatitis C and HIV disease.

Though attitudes are changing, some physicians remain reluctant to prescribe medications to treat addictive disorders or co-occurring mental health disorders. In addition, many treatment professionals still harbor negative perceptions about the use of pharmaceutical interventions. The increasing use of medications has the following significant workforce implications:

- Creates increased demand for nurses, physicians and other health care practitioners to prescribe, administer and monitor medication;
- Requires practitioners to learn to assess potential medication needs and to incorporate pharmacological interventions into treatment plans and treatment protocols; and
- Results in further rapprochement between the specialist treatment and generalist medical care systems to bridge workforce gaps when they cannot be filled through hiring. This could well manifest itself as co-location of generalist and specialist staff in both systems.

Over the next decade, the ability to use medications to treat both mental health and addictive disorders will become increasingly important. The demands on the workforce will be significant and cross-systems collaboration will be essential to make available the kinds of multi disciplinary teams necessary to effectively provide care in this environment. States and localities have varying requirements with respect to medical staffing in addictions treatment programs. Some require programs to have medical and nursing staff, while others have no such requirements. Moreover, there is wide variation in the level of medical staffing across programs even within jurisdictions. A recent national study found that only 54 percent of "programs had even a part-time physician on staff. Outside of methadone programs, less than 15 percent of programs employed a nurse" (McLellan et al., 2003). Mechanisms for recruiting and training additional physicians, nurses and other primary health care practitioners will need to be found.

Movement toward a Recovery Management Model of Care

Although substance use disorders are often chronic, conventional treatment approaches have typically used acute models of care. As Dennis, Scott and Funk (2003) note:

> Longitudinal studies have repeatedly demonstrated that addictions treatment (particularly for 90 or more days) is associated with major reductions in substance use, problems and costs to society ... However, post-discharge relapse and eventual re-admission are also the norm ...The risk of relapse does not appear to abate until 4 to 5 years of abstinence ... Retrospective and prospective treatment studies report that most clients undergo 3 to 4 episodes of care before reaching a stable state of abstinence ... In spite of this evidence of chronicity and multiple episodes of care, most ... treatment continues to be characterized as relatively self-encapsulated, serial episodes of acute treatment with post discharge aftercare typically limited to passive referrals to self-help groups.

In the past 15 years, the primary health care field has developed a new approach to the treatment and management of chronic health care disorders such as diabetes mellitus, hypertension and asthma. This approach is called "disease management." Managed care organizations have built disease management protocols into requirements for the treatment of chronic conditions, such as diabetes. Segments of the addictions treatment field are beginning to evaluate how they can apply similar models. Such models are critically important as the use of medication-assisted therapies for substance use disorders becomes more prevalent, and as the profile of the publicly-funded addictions patient/client becomes more complex, involving an increasing variety of co- morbid medical and psychiatric conditions that must be managed in concert with the substance use disorder.

The disease/recovery management concept applied to addictions treatment focuses on interventions that strengthen and extend the length of remission periods, reduce the number, intensity and duration of relapse events and quickly re-engage individuals in services at the time of relapse. Recovery management models:

- Apply new advances in scientific research and practice;
- Build upon peer-to-peer support, a practice used traditionally in the field;
- Involve individuals in the management of their own illnesses;
- Implement best practices with a professionally trained workforce, supported by trained recovery specialists;
- Use case management to ensure continuity of care;
- Place greater emphasis on the long-term recovery process as opposed to a specific treatment episode; and
- Incorporate monitoring support (e.g., check-ups) throughout treatment, using the results to guide the course of subsequent care.

States are including disease/recovery management in their substance use disorder treatment services. For example, the State of Connecticut has designated the concept of "recovery" as the overarching goal of its delivery system for mental health and addictions services. Through identified model programs, it has created Centers for Excellence in key recovery-oriented areas: outreach and engagement, cultural competency, person-centered planning, peer-run programs, core skills and supported community living. The State of Arizona has revised its Medicaid plan for addictions services to include peer-delivered recovery support through the full continuum of care.

Findings to date on the application of recovery management principles are encouraging. For example, a recent NIDA-funded study of individuals (n = 448) randomly assigned to recovery management checkups (RMCs), assessments, motivational interviewing and linkage to treatment re-entry, found that participants assigned to RMCs were significantly more likely than those in the control group to return to treatment, to return to treatment sooner and to spend more subsequent days in treatment. They were also significantly less likely to be in need of additional treatment at 24 months (Dennis et al., 2003).

Preliminary research indicates that recovery management approaches hold great promise. To the extent that States and treatment provider organizations adopt such approaches, the workforce will not only need training and support to integrate these protocols, but will also need to establish networks with a variety of traditional and non-traditional partners.

Provision of Services in Generalist and Specialist Settings

A diverse group of individuals within the addictions treatment workforce provide services in two sectors: the generalist and specialist treatment sectors. The generalist setting consists of primary health care centers and other community settings (e.g., trauma centers/emergency rooms, ob-gyn clinics, occupational medicine programs, schools with student assistance programs and student health services, welfare offices and work sites with employee assistance programs). The specialist setting is designed to treat individuals with substance use disorders. It consists of specialized services provided by not-for-profit, and for-profit organizations and by private practitioners. The vast majority of specialty addictions treatment is provided through community-based, not-for-profit agencies with public funds.

At present, the following activities are beginning to be implemented in selected generalist settings:

- Screening for alcohol and drug problems;
- Brief intervention and brief treatment for non-dependent users; and
- Referral and follow-up to the specialist treatment system for dependent users.

Historically, generalist staff have usually not screened and provided services related to substance use problems, and addictions treatment specialist staff have rarely been stationed in generalist settings to provide such services. However, changes are occurring due to a recognized need to intervene with individuals before high-risk behaviors progress to a diagnosable substance use disorder. Very few generalist setting staff have been trained in substance use disorders. They lack the knowledge to detect such problems. To help overcome these barriers, SAMHSA developed the SBIRT initiative. In FY

2006, this effort is now being implemented in nine States. An evaluation of this $30 million effort is underway, so that the field may benefit from the knowledge gained from it.

The diversity of the population with substance use problems requires the workforce to be equipped to address issues as they arise in both the generalist and specialist settings. A large segment of the population would benefit greatly from earlier detection of this illness, potentially reducing the number of individuals who would eventually require specialty treatment. However, the workforce within the generalist setting is not prepared to address this issue in a significant manner without substantially more education and training, including training related to serving those with co-occurring disorders.

The complexity of the specialist setting raises unique challenges for workforce development across both the public and private sectors. Not only do funding mechanisms and minimum staffing and care requirements vary greatly from State to State, but publicly and privately funded organizations have differing priorities, incentives, organizational cultures, philosophies, service mixes and target populations. Additionally, the workforce within the specialist setting has ongoing training needs due to changing treatment technology, staff turnover and recent initiatives to begin engaging individuals in the early stages of substance use problems through co-location or linkage with generalist settings. Cross-training of generalists and specialists is critically important. The magnitude of substance use disorders and the opportunity to leverage resources dedicated to their treatment require that the two settings work together to meet the challenges that drug and alcohol use present.

Use of Performance and Patient Outcome Measures

The addictions field is experiencing increasing demands for accountability in treatment performance. Funding entities and service providers want quantitative feedback on the benefits experienced by service recipients and on measures necessary for enhanced treatment efficiency and effectiveness. The Washington Circle Group, "a multi-disciplinary group of providers, researchers, managed care representatives and public policy makers" convened by SAMHSA in 1998 to develop a core set of performance measures for addictions treatment, has noted that "monitoring the quality and availability of alcohol and other drug services must be a central tenet of any health-related performance measurement system." The Washington Circle Group has further noted that "performance measures for alcohol and other drugs need to become an integral part of a comprehensive set of behavioral and physical health performance measures for managed care plans" (Washington Circle Group, 2005).

SAMHSA has required the collection of National Outcome Measures (NOMs) to track outcomes and performance related to treatment services funded under the Substance Abuse Prevention and Treatment Block Grant. All States are required to report by September 2007. Discretionary grantees are already reporting NOMs. NOMs track outcomes and performance across 10 domains: 1) abstinence; 2) employment/education; 3) crime and criminal justice; 4) housing stability; 5) access/capacity; 6) retention; 7) social connectedness; 8) perception of care; 9) cost-effectiveness; and 10) use of evidence-based practices. To support States in their data collection and reporting, SAMHSA will provide infrastructure and technical assistance through a new State Outcomes Measurement and Management System (SOMMS). Because the majority of addictions treatment services nationally are publicly funded, NOMs will become one of the most broadly adopted sets of outcomes/performance measures.

Nationally, across both private and public sector managed care plans, the Health Plan Employer Data and Information Set (HEDIS) is the most widely adopted package of performance measures (Washington Circle Group, 2004). Developed by the National Committee for Quality Assurance (NCQA), HEDIS is a set of standardized performance measures designed to permit reliable comparison of the performance of managed health care plans (NCQA, 2005). Until 2003, it included no performance measures related to the treatment of addictive disorders.

In February 2003, NCQA added two measures specific to substance use disorders that had been developed by the Washington Circle Group: 1) *Identification of Alcohol and Other Drug Services*, which tracks the percentage of plan members who initiate addictions treatment services and the type of service provided; and 2) *Initiation and Engagement of Alcohol and Other Drug Dependence Treatment*, which measures the percentage of plan members who receive two or more additional substance use disorder services within 30 days of initiation (NCQA, 2003).

In a report entitled *Rewarding Results: Improving the Quality of Treatment for People with Alcohol and Drug Problems,* a national policy panel headed by Jerome Jaffe, M.D., affirmed the Washington Circle Group's performance measures. However, the panel recognized that a "weak infrastructure dramatically limits the effectiveness of many basic quality improvement strategies." The panel acknowledged that "many programs are well run and provide high quality care," but pointed out that "too many are fiscally weak and unstable." The panel argued that "only in a more stable treatment system can we hope to use training to achieve significant increments in quality" (Join Together, 2003).

To begin developing a stable infrastructure upon which to build training, technology transfer and quality improvement systems, the panel report recommended that public and private funders financially reward programs with good results, such as reduced drug and alcohol use, reduced medical services utilization, reduced criminal justice system involvement and increased employment. Acknowledging the difficult truth that doing so would mean "taking patients and funds from programs with consistently poor results," the panel recognized that weaker programs would likely need to close or consolidate with other programs. However, the panel expected that under such financial incentives, "new partnerships should evolve among providers that help them preserve their viability without total merger – for example, arrangements that allow them to share specialized personnel and administrative or technology costs" (Join Together, 2003).

Commitment is required at the national, State and local levels to significantly improve the quality of addictions treatment. Such efforts would go a long way toward securing for the field the recognition and central role in health care systems that it merits. The field must play such a role to effectively address the addictions treatment needs faced within the United States.

Discrimination Associated with Addictions and the Addictions Treatment Workforce

Negative perceptions of addictions have far-reaching results that go beyond their impact on the treatment workforce. A Join Together issue paper says rampant discrimination restricts access to education, housing, employment, financial assistance and health care for people with addictions (2001). Some examples are:

- Insurance policies that deny or restrict coverage for addictions treatment;
- The Drug Free Student Aid provision of the U.S. Higher Education Act, which denies financial aid to students with a drug conviction; and
- The 1996 welfare reform provision that imposes a lifetime ban on welfare benefits for people convicted of possessing or selling drugs.

According to *The Christian Science Monitor*, experts in treatment and recovery estimate that when recovering individuals are honest about their drug histories, they will be turned down for a job 75 percent of the time (Marks, 2002). A Join Together feature article cites a California survey in which 59 percent of employers said they would never hire anyone with a felony conviction (Curley, 2002).

As noted above, discrimination also results in avoidance of treatment, often delaying care until the substance use disorder has progressed substantially and/or complex co-occurring disorders emerge or worsen. Among one million people who were identified as needing treatment and felt that they needed it but did not receive treatment, 19.6 percent reported that they did not try to access it due to the stigma associated with addictions (NSDUH, 2004b). The net result of such treatment avoidance is that individuals present to treatment later with more complicated needs. They are subsequently more costly to treat than they would have been had an intervention occurred earlier. Effectively addressing stigma around addictions could result in more timely intervention, improved outcomes and reduced health care costs.

Discrimination also affects the addictions treatment professional. Many believe that the stigma attached to addictions results in decreased funding to address workforce issues and has a detrimental effect on attracting and retaining professionals in the workforce. Addictions treatment struggles to be recognized as a field that provides vital health care for a life-threatening chronic disorder.

Implications of Current Trends

Over the past decade, trends have reflected the increasing pressures experienced by the addictions treatment workforce. Individuals entering treatment are presenting with more complex and severe disorders. Private health plan coverage of addictions treatment has declined in fixed dollars and as a percentage of overall health plan coverage over the past decade, placing increasing burdens on publicly funded treatment systems. In 1991, private insurance accounted for 24 percent of substance abuse treatment expenditures, whereas, in 2001, it accounted for only 13 percent (Mark et al., 2005). At the same time, the profile of the publicly funded addictions treatment patient/client has changed. Clinicians and programs must be prepared to address the needs of both a more severely impaired population, with problems that are more numerous and more intractable, and a less impaired population that is being referred earlier in the progression of an addictive disorder. To maintain skills that will keep pace with the rapidly changing environment, the workforce must be resilient, clinically competent and adaptable. Addressing these challenges will require ongoing knowledge and skill development at the executive, management and practitioner levels, and will also require diversification of the workforce through specialization among counselors and through the addition of a larger number of allied professionals. Specialized expertise is needed in areas such as brief treatment, medication- assisted therapies and co-occurring disorders.

II. STAKEHOLDER RECOMMENDATIONS

The Stakeholder Recommendations section summarizes the input from the diverse stakeholders, cites relevant literature and makes recommendations across major topic areas including the identity of the addictions treatment field and the challenges and opportunities it faces.

A. Infrastructure Development Priorities

Infrastructure Issues in Brief

A sound addictions treatment infrastructure ensures the availability of a qualified workforce capable of meeting the treatment and recovery needs of diverse populations. This infrastructure must include mechanisms to attract, educate, train and retain staff and to support the dynamic capacity of the treatment delivery system. The infrastructure also must include information systems that support and enhance workers' abilities to manage treatment services and ensure accountability and quality of care.

Current data indicate that more than 67,000 practitioners provide addictions treatment and related services (Harwood, 2002). By 2010, the need for addictions professionals and licensed treatment staff with graduate-level degrees is expected to increase by 35 percent (NASADAD, 2003). With anecdotal evidence already indicating a shortage of staff, more severe staffing shortages are anticipated in the near future. Exacerbating this issue is the current unmet need for treatment services. Staff workloads are high, salaries are low and employee benefits are minimal. The effects on the workforce are dramatic: staff turnover rates of nearly 20 percent and high levels of worker dissatisfaction (Knudsen et al., 2003; Gallon et al., 2003).

With treatment organizations struggling to recruit and retain staff, attracting individuals to the field to expand capacity is a challenge. A modest 10 percent increase in treatment capacity would require an additional 6,800 clinicians above the annual number currently required to replace staff leaving clinical practice (The Lewin Group, 2004). The treatment system's capacity to close the gap in alcohol and drug treatment is threatened by a lack of national occupational standards, inadequate incentives to enter the addictions treatment workforce and an absence of defined career paths.

Stakeholder Recommendations

To strengthen the addictions treatment infrastructure, stakeholders made the following recommendations:

1. **Create career paths for the treatment and recovery workforce and adopt national core competency standards.**

Career paths provide structure for organizations and individuals in the workforce and identify potential opportunities for career advancement. Additionally, career paths help individuals understand that they are part of a profession, validating not only training and academic credentials, but also time in the field and prior experience. Career paths also support the retention of competent professionals, help to identify the range of managerial, supervisory and other professional options available to those entering the field, enable workers to plan their own professional development and set career goals and give recognition and status to individuals progressing along a track to higher-level positions.

Competency standards articulate expectations of professional practice and ensure that individuals holding a specific type of position have the same basic core knowledge, skill and/or ability. While every State has a credentialing process and most States have an entry-level counselor credential (NASADAD, 2003), credentialing standards differ among States and, within a few States, there is more than one credentialing organization. In addition, there are no uniformly adopted credentialing standards for social workers, psychologists, nurses, physicians and other professionals who practice in the addictions treatment and recovery field. National core competency standards for addictions treatment professionals have not been adopted.

Creating career paths that incorporate core competencies provides credibility to the field, and professional development and advancement opportunities for those wishing to enter the workforce.

2. Foster network development.

A study of the national addictions treatment infrastructure found that the organizational and administrative infrastructures of many addictions programs were inadequate and unstable (McLellan et al., 2003). In fact, of the 175 drug and alcohol treatment programs included in the study, 15 percent had either closed or stopped providing addictions treatment services. Additionally, 29 percent had been taken over or "reorganized" under a different administrative structure.

As the field faces agency closures, particularly among smaller treatment providers, networks represent an important mechanism for ensuring agency viability and service availability. In addition, networks can provide career paths for addictions professionals and potential staffing pools for member organizations.

3. Provide technical assistance to enhance the capacity to use information technology.

Many treatment organizations lag behind their counterparts in the health care industry with regard to the ability to access and use information technology. A recent study, for example, found that 20 percent of 175 counseling centers surveyed had no information systems, e-mail or even voice-mail (McLellan et al., 2003). Further, although 50 percent of the treatment programs studied had a computerized information system available to administrative staff, these systems did not support the provision or monitoring of care. The systems were, instead, dedicated exclusively to billing or administrative record keeping.

Widely available technologies to support clinical and administrative services could alleviate many workforce challenges if they were broadly adopted by the addictions treatment field. Technology offers at least three important service opportunities for patients/clients and staff: (1) management of clinical practices and administrative paperwork; (2) staff participation in on line learning; and (3) provider on-line patient counseling, i.e., e-therapy. The ability of providers to access and use computer technology effectively can mean the difference between whether some people—especially patients in rural areas, the physically disabled and other underserved populations—receive treatment or not (New Freedom Commission, 2003).

B. Leadership and Management Priorities

Leadership and Management Issues in Brief

The addictions treatment field has undergone significant changes in recent years, including a greater emphasis on accountability, patient-centered care and best practices. These changes place significant demands on the workforce, particularly leaders and managers in the field who have primary responsibility for ensuring that organizations have systems in place to support and manage the achievement of positive treatment outcomes.

The extent of the leadership and management issues in the addictions treatment field is evidenced by a 53 percent turnover rate in 2002 for program managers and directors (McLellan et al., 2003). The aging of program managers further compounds the need to develop a new generation of leaders.

Greater use of best practices has also placed new demands on staff supervisors and managers who need the knowledge and skills to reinforce new practices. Management must also provide detailed expectations of supervisors' roles and responsibilities as technology transfer agents to make the adoption of evidence-based practices successful (Heathfield, 2004).

Training alone is not adequate to ensure full and effective application of practices and their sustainability over time. In cases where practice differs from past methods, intensive supervision is essential to ensure that technology transfer occurs. As noted in *The Change Book*, "too often brief flurries of training alone are thought to be sufficient in bringing about lasting change. The results are usually short-lived alterations in practice followed by discouragement and a return to familiar but less effective ways of doing things" (ATTC, 2004). A technology transfer strategy is required to ensure effective adoption of evidence-based best practices. Technology transfer "involves creating a mechanism by which a desired change is accepted, incorporated and reinforced at all levels of an organization or system" (ATTC, 2004). For best practices to be adopted, leadership and management must develop a technology transfer strategy to ensure long- lasting organizational change.

Stakeholder Recommendations

To address leadership and management issues in the addictions treatment workforce, stakeholders made the following recommendations:

1. **Develop, deliver and sustain training for treatment and recovery support supervisors, who serve as the technology transfer agents for the latest research and best practices.**

Scientific advances and the emphasis on patient/client outcomes have heightened the need for well-trained, highly skilled and dedicated clinical supervisors. More than 80 percent of these early-career staff identified clinical supervision as having the greatest value in their professional development (NAADAC, 2003). However, as stakeholders pointed out, individuals are often promoted to supervisory positions without management training or specifically defined roles.

Clinical supervisors are critical to sustaining and developing staff competencies and must become a key focus of professional development efforts. Further, training for clinical supervisors must be based on a set of core competencies. Given the increased attention being placed on patient/client outcomes, the role of clinical supervisors as technology transfer agents is vital. Training specifically targeting recovery support services supervisors is also necessary.

2. **Develop, deliver and sustain leadership and management development initiatives.**

Leadership and management practices impact all aspects of the organization: fiscal, clinical, administrative and human resources. A study (Knudsen et al., 2003) suggests good management practices that can improve staff retention and reduce turnover. These include:

- Increased job autonomy;
- Recognition and reward for strong job performance; and
- Establishing a work environment that supports creativity and innovation.

Many changes have occurred since the current generation of leaders entered the field. As co- morbid medical and mental health disorders are identified with increasing frequency among those served, the provision of treatment has become more complex, requiring the participation of multiple disciplines. Science has taken on a prominent role as the basis for addictions practices and there is a greater focus on outcomes and accountability. As the addictions treatment field grows, the need for effective leadership has never been greater.

Most organizations that provide addictions treatment services do not have a coordinated plan to manage existing and future gaps in leadership. Required leadership and business management skills have become more complex and include strategic planning; fiscal planning; an understanding of Federal, State and local policies; and contracting, communications (e.g., public speaking), collaboration skills and mentoring.

C. Recruitment Priorities

Recruitment Issues in Brief

The ability to maintain an adequate addictions treatment workforce is threatened by the difficulty in recruiting staff. The Bureau of Labor Statistics estimates that there will be 3,000 unfilled positions for addictions counselors by the year 2010 (Landis et al., 2002). Concurrently, as noted above, NASADAD projects that the need for treatment staff with graduate degrees will increase by 35% by 2010 (NASADAD, 2003). Another study reports that 5,000 new counselors will be needed each year to replace those leaving the workforce (The Lewin Group, 1994). In addition, stakeholders offer anecdotal information indicating that staffing shortages exist at every level of the workforce. Demographic changes, particularly the aging of the current workforce, are expected to worsen these shortages over the next decade.

Innovative and comprehensive recruitment strategies are needed, and must accommodate the dynamic nature of the treatment field, including increased demand related to new types of funding for treatment services, the need to keep pace with scientific advances, staff turnover and required training time for staff. Recruitment efforts must also address the underlying conditions that make people reluctant to enter the addictions treatment workforce: low salaries, minimal benefits, negative public perceptions of the field, high caseloads, patients' increasingly complex health care needs, low professional status and stressful working conditions (Knudsen and Gabriel, 2003).

Treatment agencies compete with other sectors of the economy that often pay higher wages and place fewer demands on workers' time. The need for staff with higher levels of education and training is greater now than it was even a few years ago due to the (1) increasing complexity of the patient/client population entering treatment and (2) scientific advances in treatment. The pool of trained workers is failing to keep up with demand. Compounding these issues is the limited supply of new workers. Between 2000 and 2030, for example, the total population of working-age individuals (18 to 64 years) is projected to grow by only 16 percent (Scanlon, 2001).

Staff recruitment is therefore taking on greater urgency in the addictions treatment field. Unquestionably, the issues exacerbating staff recruitment problems are complex and difficult to resolve. The field is challenged with developing creative strategies that address these recruitment issues and must work in partnership with educational institutions, Federal and State agencies, the public health care system, the media and others to develop and implement effective strategies.

Key strategies should be developed for increasing the diversity of the addictions treatment workforce so that it more closely reflects the patient/client population. As Figure 3 (below) shows, there are discrepancies between the demographics of the addictions treatment staff and the addictions treatment patients/clients. Clinicians tend to be White females over the age of 45, while most patients/clients are younger males with more diverse racial and ethnic backgrounds. The addictions treatment workforce must become more diverse and culturally competent at all levels to better serve the patient/client population (Kaplan, 2003).

Stakeholder Recommendations

Stakeholders made the following recommendations:

1. Expand recruitment of health care professionals in addictions medicine.

The tremendous growth over the past two decades in the availability of medications in substance use disorder treatment, and the increasingly complicated medical conditions that the patient/client population brings to treatment, reaffirm the need for more nurses, physicians and psychiatrists in specialty treatment. Few programs, other than those that offer methadone as an adjunct to treatment, have nurses on staff and just over half employ physicians (McLellan et al., 2003).

Some of the boundaries that have traditionally separated specialty addictions and generalist medicine need to become substantially more porous in order to permit the development of strong workforces and truly responsive care systems. Generally, strategies need to be developed to attract larger numbers of physicians to addictions medicine and to encourage larger numbers of nurses and medical social workers to obtain addictions certification. As Figure 4 shows, a relatively small percentage of physicians, nurses and other health professionals obtain addictions credentials or self-identify as an addictions specialist.

	Clinicians	Patients
Age	Average age: 45-50	50% between ages 25-44
Race	70-90% Non-Hispanic Whites	60% Non-Hispanic Whites
Gender	50-70% Female	70% Male Admissions

Source: Kaplan, 2003; SAMHSA, 2002.

Figure 3. Demographics of the Workforce.

Recruitment strategies need to begin with professional associations, credentialing bodies and the institutions of higher learning and teaching hospitals where physicians, nurses, social workers, psychologists and other allied professionals are trained.

Physicians, psychiatrists, nurses and other medical providers must be recruited within the generalist setting to provide a variety of care, including SBIRT, primary health care and mental health services.

Discipline	Workforce Size	Certified Addictions Specialists
Primary care	700,000	2,790 ASAM certified
Psychiatry	30,000	1,067 addictions psychiatrists
Clinical Psychology	69,800	950 APA substance abuse certified
Social Work	300,000	29,400*
Nursing	2,200,000	4,100*
Physician assistant	27,500	185*
Marriage/family therapy	50,000	2,500*

* Self-described addictions specialist
Source: IOM, 1997.

Figure 4. Number of Practitioners and Certified Addictions Specialists, by Health Care Discipline.

2. Improve student recruitment with educational institutions, focusing on under-represented groups.

Student recruitment, at various age levels, is needed to expand the addictions treatment workforce. Educational efforts should begin as early as elementary school, continuing through middle school and high school. Recruitment activities should begin in high school and continue through postgraduate education.

In particular, recruitment should focus on students with diverse racial and ethnic backgrounds and males to achieve a greater balance between the treatment clinicians and patients/clients.

Healthy People 2010 maintains that "increasing the number of minority health professionals is . . . a partial solution to improving access to care" (DHHS, 2000). Paraphrasing one of the key conclusions of the IOM report, *In the Nation's Compelling Interest: Ensuring Diversity in the Health Care Workforce* (2004), IOM member Brian Smedley stated, "Part of a comprehensive strategy to reduce health disparities is to increase diversity in the health care professions, which will lead to improved access to care, greater patient satisfaction and reduced cultural and linguistic barriers" (Levin, 2004).

3. Employ marketing strategies to attract workers to the addictions treatment field.

Nursing and other professions have made effective use of the media to recruit workers. For example, an intensive multi-year campaign to attract individuals to nursing was implemented in 2002 (Johnson & Johnson, 2003). One year later, after years of declining enrollment, nursing schools began to experience an increase in the number of applicants and in enrollment.

The addictions treatment field should adopt similar strategies with the anticipation of seeing comparable results. Using basic principles of health communication and social marketing, the field should develop targeted, consumer-centered messages through deliberate placement of advertising designed to reach specific audience segments, including young people and minorities, to create diverse applicant pools. All media options and recruitment channels (e.g., employee referrals, job fairs, classified advertising, links with educational institutions and online job sites) should be explored.

Stakeholders pointed out that there are populations that recruitment efforts should target. It will be critically important to recruit younger individuals who are interested in finding a long-term career path in addictions treatment. Over the long term it is through young persons who elect to make addictions treatment a career that the field will develop most fully as a unique profession. Second- career professionals, while potentially having a shorter career span, bring maturity, broad life and work experience to the field that is extremely valuable. Those in recovery and their family members have long brought unique, first-hand experience, passion and perspective to the field. They represent an immense pool of potential workers whose talents would provide an immeasurable benefit to the field. While such individuals already represent a significant segment of the addictions treatment workforce, the field has barely begun to tap this rich resource.

4. Continue efforts to reduce the stigma associated with working in addictions treatment.

Stigma devalues addictions treatment as a meaningful career and reduces the size of the prospective labor pool, making staff recruitment difficult. Workforce recruitment efforts must overcome the stigmatization of the addictions treatment field. Other health professions, like nursing, have implemented successful initiatives to address stigmatization and its negative impacts. The success of stigma reduction efforts has instilled the nursing profession with a more positive self-image and shown nurses to be a valuable and necessary national resource. The nursing profession has approached the issue of stigma and its workforce crisis in a variety of ways (Nevidjon and Erickson, 2001). It has:

- Worked to define and distinguish the profession through research, education, and clinical service;
- Engaged professional nursing associations as advocates to gain support and recognition;
- Obtained support from professional colleagues (e.g., doctors); and
- Challenged the media to present positive and true images of the nursing profession (Donley et al., 2002).

Although negative images and stigma associated with nursing have not disappeared entirely and a nursing shortage still exists, progress has been made. A study by Bacon, MacKenzie and McKendrick (2000), for example, found that nurses are now viewed as well-educated, independent thinkers who play a key role within a high-tech medical world. This improved image has enabled the field to recruit more young people and career-minded professionals. These strategies provide examples of what could be accomplished in the addictions treatment field.

D. Addictions Education and Accreditation Priorities

Education and Accreditation Issues in Brief

Academic training is fundamental to developing a quality workforce and to providing quality care. Although progress has been made in raising academic standards in addictions studies programs to the level of programs in other health care disciplines, several serious gaps remain.

A significant problem is the lack of education and training on substance use disorders for primary health care and other health and human services professionals. The National Center on Addictions and Substance Abuse (CASA) at Columbia University reported that 94 percent of primary care physicians and 40 percent of pediatricians, when presented with a person with a substance use disorder, failed to diagnose the problem properly (CASA, 2000). If similar studies were available for other health professionals (e.g., nurses, psychologists, pharmacists, social workers, dentists), the results would likely be similar. The primary reason for health professionals' failure to diagnose substance use disorders is a lack of knowledge about the disease. Curricula in most health education programs and professional schools either inadequately address substance use disorders or exclude discussion of them altogether.

New demands are being placed on the higher education system as the need for academic training grows within the addictions treatment field. Historically, training for addictions treatment tended to resemble an apprentice model. This model emphasizes experience over formal education. An apprentice model can best be described as training in which the majority of knowledge, skills and ability to practice are imparted through supervision. With the need to treat and manage complex patients/clients and implement evidence-based practices in the workplace, the call for more formal education to complement supervision is changing the workforce culture. Increasingly, States are finding the need to require formal education through credentialing and licensure standards (SAMHSA, 2005).

Colleges and universities rely on a variety of standards to develop curricula, rather than one set of national competencies. Although efforts have been made to establish national academic accreditation standards for addictions studies, they have not been adopted. Program accreditation would provide recognition and demonstrate an ongoing commitment to quality education.

Presently, 442 colleges and universities across the country offer addictions studies programs. Eighteen percent are at the graduate level, 13 percent are at the undergraduate level and 69 percent are at the associate level (Taleff, 2003). Anecdotally, information from stakeholders suggests that tremendous variation exists among these academic programs with regard to level of course difficulty, use of evidence-based materials, quality of faculty and ability to prepare students for clinical practice. Additionally, the relevance of coursework and its relationship to research depends greatly on faculty members' abilities to stay current on recently completed and ongoing research.

The changing demographics of the Nation demand a multi-cultural and multi-lingual workforce. Although enrollment remains at record high levels for traditional college-age students, those under 25 years old (Jamieson et al., 2001), data are not available about the number of racial and ethnic minorities enrolled in addictions studies programs, or the progress that has been made to increase minority enrollment.

Stakeholder Recommendations

To improve the academic caliber of education programs for the addictions treatment field, stakeholders made the following recommendations:

1. **Include training on addictions as part of education programs for primary health care and for other health and human service professions (e.g., physicians, nurses, psychologists and social workers).**

Primary care physicians and other health professionals frequently are the first point of contact in the health care system, yet they often do not recognize substance use disorders. Failure to diagnose and refer patients with substance use disorders occurs, in large part, because of the lack of academic or other training related to substance use disorders. A national survey of residency program directors in seven medical specialties revealed that only 56 percent of the residency programs surveyed had a required curriculum in preventing and treating alcohol and substance use disorders. The most common barriers to providing training were a lack of time (58%), a lack of faculty expertise (37%) and a lack of institutional support (32%). According to the authors, education programs can be improved by integrating training on addictions into existing residency structures, increasing faculty knowledge and including more questions related to treatment on board examinations (Isaacson et al., 2000).

Similar programs would benefit social workers. Many clinical social workers are eligible to practice in the addictions treatment field as a result of their social work license, but may lack the specialty education and training that would permit them to provide the most effective care. A 2000 survey of the members of the National Association of Social Workers by the Practice Research Network (PRN) Project found that only 38 percent of members had completed formal coursework in substance use disorder treatment during their academic programs, and 87 percent indicated that they held no certification in the treatment of substance use disorders (NASW PRN, 2001).

2. Call for the use of national addictions core competencies as the basis of curricula.

Educational curricula must be based on solid research and on a unified national set of core competencies to prepare a workforce that is both knowledgeable and skilled. Educational institutions use a number of standards when developing curricula. These standards include the IC&RC twelve core functions; the International Coalition for Addictions Studies Education (INCASE) standards; the NAADAC Certification Standards; and SAMHSA's *Technical Assistance Publication 21 (TAP 21) Addiction Counseling Competencies: The Knowledge, Skills and Atti*tudes of Professional Practice (SAMHSA, 2002).

The lack of consistency in academic curricula works to the detriment of the field. Many treatment professionals and organizations agree that TAP 21 should be the basis for curriculum development. TAP 21 is designed to impart the knowledge, skills and attitudes for achieving and practicing addictions counseling competencies.

3. Support the development and adoption of national accreditation standards for addictions education programs.

Academic accreditation standards for addictions studies programs need to be developed, adopted and supported. There is no uniform national programmatic structure nor are there associated standards for addictions studies despite the existence of 442 addictions studies programs across the United States. Little is known about the quality of these programs and how they prepare future practitioners.

Academic accreditation standards should be adopted to improve the quality and standing of addictions education programs. Educators in addictions studies expressed the feeling that their programs were given "second class" status by their institutions. Accreditation has advantages for educators as well as students. Educators gain access to a network of other accredited programs for sharing best practices and professional knowledge. Faculty members participate in peer review processes. Students benefit from an enriched environment for learning and greater ease in transitioning credits from one accredited school to another.

4. **Encourage national and State boards for the health professions to have at least 10 percent of licensing examination questions pertain to addictions.**

The core curriculum in the health professions is strongly influenced by licensing examinations and certification requirements. If items on the treatment of addictions were included in the licensing and certification examinations, the topic of addictions would receive more emphasis in the core curriculum of each discipline in the field (Haack and Adger, 2002).

State addictions treatment authorities should work with licensing bodies to ensure that 10% of licensing questions pertain to addictions. To accomplish this, they will also need to work with institutions of higher education, to encourage development of curricula that prepare future professionals to address addictions.

5. **Support academic programs in Historically Black Colleges and Universities (HBCUs), Hispanic Serving Institutions, Tribal Colleges and Universities and other minority- serving institutions.**

Nationally, racial and ethnic minorities are projected to grow from 28 percent of the population in 2000 to nearly 40 percent by 2030 (Dochterman and Grace, 2001). The multicultural composition of the population requires that greater attention be given to diversifying the workforce. A significant disparity already exists between clinicians and patients/clients in the addictions treatment field. Providing support for educational programs targeting racial and ethnic minorities will ultimately result in more graduates who will become part of the treatment workforce.

Academic programs that support racial and ethnic minority students offer great promise for addressing unmet health care needs. Initiatives supporting curriculum development, internships, apprenticeships, loan forgiveness and scholarships at academic institutions that serve minority populations would provide a mechanism to increase the diversity of the workforce and provide care in underserved areas (DHHS/HRSA, 2004).

6. **Develop college and university courses on health services research and its application; and systematically disseminate research findings to academic institutions.**

One of the greatest challenges for the addictions treatment field is the dissemination and institutionalization of evidence-based practices. NIDA and NIAAA have conducted considerable research in substance use disorders. Systematic mechanisms are needed to disseminate research findings to academic institutions and to ensure that the most current research informs educational practices.

Implementing evidence-based practices requires a workforce trained to understand how to find and use new knowledge. As clearly noted in the IOM report *Crossing the Quality Chasm* (2001), clinical education needs to include courses on evidence-based practices and on learning how to access, understand and use research. Therefore, addictions studies programs at colleges and universities must include courses that teach students about research and how to apply it in practice.

E. Retention Priorities

Retention Issues in Brief

Nearly 70 percent (67.8%) of addictions treatment staff have worked with their current employer for five years or less (Harwood, 2002). Data from the University of Georgia National Treatment Center Study indicate an average annual turnover rate of 18.5 percent among addictions treatment counselors. This rate far exceeds the national average of 11 percent across all occupations and is significantly higher than the average annual turnover rates for teachers (13%) and nurses (12%), occupations traditionally known to have high staff turnover (Knudsen et al., 2003).

When retention rates are low and turnover is high, facility operations and patient/client care are compromised. Low salaries contribute to high turnover. Salaries of individuals working in the addictions treatment field are not competitive with those of other health professionals in equivalent job categories. Figure 5 provides information on the median annual earnings for addictions treatment counselors and other health and social service providers by occupation in 2000.

The U.S. Department of Labor reports that in 2000 the median income for addictions treatment and behavioral disorder counselors was $28,510. As of 2000, the mean annual salary for all addictions treatment counselors in the United States was $30,100. The region with the most counselors (mid-Atlantic) had the highest mean annual salary at $34,433 per year. While the mean annual salaries for addictions treatment counselors are comparatively low across the regions, the cost of living varies greatly by region. In many regions, salaries place many workers at bare subsistence. Additionally, a survey of addictions treatment counselors found that 30 percent had no medical coverage, 40 percent had no dental coverage and 55 percent were not covered for substance use or mental health services (Galfano, 2004).

A 2003 study of individuals in the addictions treatment workforce found that the most prevalent recommendation for retaining staff was increasing salaries (Knudsen and Gabriel, 2003). In addition, other financial incentives such as bonuses and performance awards aid in retention. Employees who perceive that their organizations provide them with more rewarding and supportive environments are more likely to be committed to the organization.

Private sector research also suggests that management practices and organizational commitments that (1) increase job autonomy and accountability for workers, (2) support creativity and new ideas and (3) provide non-tangible rewards linked to performance may improve addictions workforce retention (Knudsen et al., 2003). According to research in the public sector, good management practices that offer employee training, reduce paperwork, increase individual recognition, promote career growth and improve the physical work environment enhance retention (Knudsen and Gabriel, 2003). Creating a work environment that values and empowers all employees is vital.

Maintaining a stable workforce is the goal of every profession. Such stability helps ensure continuity, quality of care and a positive work environment. Turnover is minimized when individuals experience a high level of job satisfaction and are committed to staying in the profession. Low salaries, lack of career paths, insufficient mentorship programs, inadequate staff supervision, personnel shortages and large caseloads contribute to staff turnover and job discontent in the addictions treatment field.

The negative impact and costs of employee turnover are well documented. In testimony before the Senate Committee on Health, Education, Labor and Pensions, William J. Scanlon, Director of Health Care Issues at the

Government Accountability Office (GAO), discussed the problem of turnover in the nursing profession (Scanlon, 2001). Many of the issues Scanlon raised also pertain to the addictions treatment workforce. Specifically, Scanlon identified the following costs related to staff turnover:

- Time and expense of recruitment, selection and training of new staff;
- Inefficiencies related to entry of new staff;
- Decreased group morale and productivity; and
- Disrupted continuity of patient care.

Occupation	Median Annual Earnings ($)	Occupation	Median Annual Earnings ($)
Rehabilitation counselors	24,450	Medical and public health social workers	34,790
Mental health counselors	27,570	Educational, vocational and school counselors	42,110
Substance abuse and behavioral disorder counselors	28,510	Registered nurses	44,480
Licensed practical and vocational nurses	29,440	Psychologists (clinical, counseling and school)	48,320
Mental health and substance abuse social workers	30,170	Physician assistants	61,910
Child, family and school social workers	31,470	Family and general practitioners	130,000*
Marriage and family therapists	34,660	Psychiatrists	130,000*

Source: U.S. Department of Labor, 2003 and, when indicated by an asterisk (*), the American Medical Association

Figure 5. Median Annual Earnings of Community and Social Service Counselors and Selected Behavioral Health Professionals in 2000.

Retention efforts must be creative, innovative and address underlying reasons that cause individuals to quit their jobs or leave the field. Career path development, training on clinical supervision, leadership and management development and marketing of the field have been discussed earlier in this report and are potential retention strategies.

Stakeholder Recommendations

Stakeholders made the following additional recommendations to develop a multi-faceted retention strategy to improve workforce retention:

1. Identify and disseminate best practices in staff retention.

National leadership should be provided regarding the identification and dissemination of best practices related to salary structure and benefits, financial incentives, continuing education, alternative work schedules, mentoring, employee wellness practices and professional advancement. Dissemination of practices to State Directors, providers, ATTCs and professional and trade associations within the addictions treatment field should be a major priority.

As the field develops a multi-faceted strategy for workforce retention, it is recommended that SAMHSA identify and disseminate to the States best practices related to workforce compensation and financial incentives and support strategic planning needed to implement a national workforce retention effort.

Anecdotal evidence indicates that recruitment and retention problems associated with faculty for addictions studies programs are just as severe as those seen in the rest of the workforce. (At the present time, adequate data are not available on the academic workforce.) The challenges involved in recruiting faculty for addictions studies programs in turn make it increasingly difficult to recruit, develop and certify degreed treatment professionals. As part of a multi-faceted strategy to recruit addictions program faculty, experienced treatment professionals who are at risk of leaving the field should be offered the opportunity to participate in specially designed accelerated degree programs (i.e., Master's or Doctorate) or other training enabling them to become addictions treatment faculty at institutions of higher learning.

2. Address substance misuse and relapse within the workforce.

While all professions employ individuals in recovery, the addictions treatment field is unusual in the proportion of its workforce that is in recovery. The addictions treatment workforce is unique in that many of the recovering individuals among its ranks work in the same health care system through which they received treatment.

To date, little attention has been given to the issue of substance misuse and relapse in the workforce. The ATTCs, in partnership with clinicians, treatment providers, States and other stakeholders, can lead the development of training that recognizes and addresses substance misuse and relapse within the workforce. Training areas should include, but not be limited to, strengthening Employee Assistance Programs (EAPs), wellness programs and health insurance and disability policies. Such training would target supervisors, human resource managers, the general provider workforce and State/Territory agency staff.

Stakeholders recommended that existing programs serving professionals working in the addictions treatment field be identified, and that national, State and local certification boards or professional societies for addictions treatment professionals explore development of peer education and support programs for impaired professionals in the addictions treatment field.

Relapse within the addictions treatment workforce presents the field with significant challenges. However, the development of relapse prevention strategies, relevant policies and procedures and impaired professional and peer education programs would provide tools to respond systematically and effectively to this challenge.

F. Study Priorities

Study Issues in Brief

To date, studies on the addictions treatment workforce have been limited in number and scope. A number of ATTCs have conducted surveys of the treatment workforce (Knudsen and Gabriel, 2003; Gallon et al., 2003). The surveys, which differ in methodology, focus on issues such as academic training and professional experience, recruitment and retention, compensation, treatment models, training interests and employee satisfaction. While informative, such studies do not yield sufficient data to guide the development of the addictions treatment workforce.

Addictions treatment would benefit from research data that show the relationship between the education, training and demographic characteristics of treatment professionals and patient/client outcomes. These research findings will enable the field to make informed decisions about professional development and improved practices.

Stakeholder Recommendations

Stakeholders identified three topics as priorities:

1. **Conduct studies that examine the relationships among level of education, type of education, training and treatment outcomes.**

Minimal research currently exists on the impact of education and training on treatment outcomes.

Health services research on this topic could provide valuable information to the field by focusing on questions such as:

- Do some types of training produce better treatment outcomes than others?
- What is the relationship between a clinician's education and treatment outcomes?
- Is experiential or academic training of greater value to treatment outcomes?

2. **Conduct studies that examine the relationships among clinician and patient/client cultural, demographic and other characteristics, therapeutic alliance and treatment outcomes.**

The disparity in age, gender, race and ethnicity between clinicians and patients/clients has led to increased concerns about the impact of these differences on therapeutic alliance (the relationship that develops between a patient/client and a clinician) and treatment outcomes.

However, little substantive research is available on the effects of an addictions treatment professional's demographic, cultural background and other characteristics on patient/client treatment outcomes.

Health services research is needed to address questions such as:

- Are cultural, demographic and other characteristics of clinicians relevant to improving therapeutic alliance and/or treatment outcomes? If so, which ones?
- Do learned cultural competency skills improve therapeutic alliance and/or treatment outcomes?
- Are treatment professionals in recovery more effective?
- Does gender matching affect treatment outcomes? If so, how?

3. **Conduct studies that explore questions related to the characteristics of clinicians that enhance therapeutic alliance and outcomes.**

In the past two decades, a number of studies investigating the role of therapeutic alliance in drug treatment have been published (Meier et al., 2005). This body of literature supports the fact that the relationship skills of the clinician are important in improving patient/client outcomes. Another factor that may significantly impact therapeutic alliance is the recovery status of the clinician. Little research has been performed on the relationship between clinician recovery status, therapeutic alliance and outcomes. Therefore, the extent to which the recovery status of clinicians is associated with an effective therapeutic alliance, client satisfaction and positive outcomes is not well known. As the field strives to improve patient/client outcomes and enhance the skills of its workforce, answers to questions such as the following would provide valuable information:

- What skills are needed to build a therapeutic alliance?
- Can training improve a practitioner's ability to build a therapeutic alliance?
- What training methods are most effective?
- Is the recovery status of the clinician correlated with the quality of therapeutic alliance?
- Do the philosophy and nature of interventions employed by recovering and non- recovering clinicians vary?
- Is there a correlation between clinician recovery status and client outcomes?

CONCLUSION

This report summarizes current and emerging issues confronting the treatment workforce. The report also provides recommendations developed by stakeholders and Federal partners. They are directed at a variety of organizations, including Federal and State entities, national trade associations, credentialing and licensing bodies and academic institutions.

Recognizing the complex nature of the challenges facing the addictions treatment field, stakeholders offered a multi-faceted approach to workforce development that addressed both short-term needs and the long-term viability of the field.

REFERENCES

Addiction Technology Transfer Center Network (ATTC), *The Change Book: A Blueprint for Technology Transfer (Second Edition)*, (Kansas City, MO: ATTC, 2004).

Annie E. Casey Foundation, *The Unsolved Challenge of System Reform: The Condition of the Frontline Human Services Workforce*, (Baltimore, MD: Annie E. Casey Foundation, 2003).

Bacon, K; MacKenzie, KE; McKendrick, JH. "Tomorrow's Nurses?" *Nursing Standard*, 14(32), 2000, 31.

Center on Addictions and Substance Abuse (CASA), *Missed Opportunity: National Survey of Primary Care Physicians and Patients on Substance Abuse*, (New York: CASA, Columbia University, 2000).

Centers for Disease Control and Prevention (CDC), *HIV/AIDS Surveillance Report: Cases of HIV and AIDS in the United States, 2002*, (Atlanta, GA: CDC, 2002a).

Centers for Disease Control and Prevention (CDC), *Viral Hepatitis and Injection Drug Users*, (Atlanta, GA: CDC, 2002b).

Corrigan, PW; Steiner, L; McCracken, SG; Blaser, B; Barr, M. "Strategies for Disseminating Evidence-based Practices to Staff Who Treat People With Serious Mental Illness," *Psychiatric Services*, 52(12), 2001, 1598-1606.

Curley, B. "Discrimination Against People in Recovery Rampant, Advocates Say," *Join Together Online*, 2002, Online, <http://www.jointogether.org/sa/news/features/reader/0,1854,553416,00.html>, Oct. 2004.

Dennis, M; Scott, CK; Funk, R. "An Experimental Evaluation of Recovery Management Checkups (RMC) for People with Chronic Substance Use Disorders," *Evaluation and Program Planning*, 26(3), 2003, 339-352.

Department of Health and Human Services (DHHS), "Access to Quality Health Care Services," *Healthy People 2010: Understanding and Improving Health*, 2nd ed., (Washington, DC: U.S. Government Printing Office, 2000), Online, <http://www.healthypeople.gov/Document/HTML/Volume1/01Access.htm>, March 2005, 20.

Department of Health and Human Services/Health Resources and Services Administration (DHHS/HRSA), "Optimizing the Impact of the National Health Service Corps," (Rockville, MD: DHHS, 2004).

Dochterman, JM; Grace, HK. "Overview: Diversity in Nursing," *Nursing*, 2001, 480-482.

Donley, R; Flaherty, MJ; Sarsfield, E; Taylor, L; Maloni, H; Flanagan, E. "What Does the Nurse Reinvestment Act Mean to You?" *Online Journal of Issues in Nursing*, 2002, *Online*, <http://www.nursingworld.org/ojin/topic14/tpc14_5.htm>, January 2005.

Drug Enforcement Administration (DEA), *Illegal Drug Price and Purity Report*, (Washington, DC: DEA, 2003).

Drug Enforcement Administration (DEA), "Drug Trafficking in the United States," (Washington, DC: DEA, 2001), *Online*, <www.dea.gov/concern/drug_trafficking>, Oct. 2004.

Galfano, S. "2004 Addictions Treatment Professional Career and Salary Survey," *Counselor: The Magazine for Addictions Professionals*, Vol. 5, 2004, 24-29.

Gallon, S; Gabriel, R; Knudsen, J. "The Toughest Job You'll Ever Love: A Pacific Northwest Treatment Workforce Survey," *Journal of Substance Abuse Treatment* 24(3), 2003, 183-196.

Gfroerer, JC; Penne, MA; Pemberton, MR; Folsom, RE. "The Aging Baby Boom Cohort and Future Prevalence of Substance Abuse," *Substance Use by Older Adults: Estimates of Future Impact on the Treatment System*, (Rockville, MD: DHHS, SAMHSA, 2002).

Grant, BF; Stinson, FS; Dawson, DA; Chou, SP; Dufour, MC; Compton, W; Pickering, RP & Kaplan, K. "Prevalence and Co-occurrence of Substance Use Disorders and Independent Mood and Anxiety Disorders: Results From the National Epidemiologic Survey on Alcohol and Related Conditions," *Archives of General Psychiatry*, 61(8), 2004, 807-816.

Haack, MR; Adger, H. "Strategic Plan for Interdisciplinary Faculty Development: Arming the Nation's Workforce for a New Approach to Substance Use Disorders," *Journal of the Association for Medical Education and Research in Substance Abuse*, 23(3), Supplement, (Providence, RI: AMERSA, 2002), 1-21.

Hager, MA; Brudney, JL. *Volunteer Management Practices and Retention of Volunteers*, (Washington, DC: The Urban Institute, 2004).

Harwood, HJ. "Survey on Behavioral Health Workplace," *Frontlines: Linking Alcohol Services Research and Practice*, (Bethesda, MD: NIAAA, 2002).

Heathfield, SM. "Ten Tips to Make Training Work," 2004, *Online*, <http://humanresources.about.com/library/weekly/aa081400a.htm>, Oct. 2004.

Hennessy, KD. *SAMHSA's Science to Services Initiative and Expansion of the National Registry of Effective Practices and Programs (NREPP)*,

Presentation to 14th Anniversary Conference on SMHA Services Research, Program Evaluation and Policy, 2004, *Online*, <http://www.nri-inc.org/Conference/Conf04/Presentations/Hennessy.pdf>, Jan. 2005.

Institute of Medicine (IOM), *Improving the Quality of Health Care for Mental and Substance-Use Conditions: Quality Chasm Series,* (Washington, DC: National Academies Press, 2006).

Institute of Medicine (IOM), *In the Nation's Compelling Interest: Ensuring Diversity in the Health Care Workforce*, (Washington, DC: National Academies Press, 2004).

Institute of Medicine (IOM), *Crossing the Quality Chasm: A New Health System for the 21st Century*, (Washington, DC: National Academies Press, 2001).

Institute of Medicine (IOM), *Managing Managed Care: Quality Improvements in Behavioral Health*, (Washington, DC: National Academies Press, 1997).

Isaacson, JH; Fleming, M; Kraus, M; Kahn, R; Mundt, M. "A National Survey of Training in Substance Use Disorders in Residency Programs," *Journal of Studies on Alcohol*, 61(6), 2000, 912-915.

Jamieson, A; Curry, A; Martinez, G. "School Enrollment-Social and Economic Characteristics of Students," *Current Population Reports,* (Washington, DC: U.S. Census Bureau, 2001).

Johnson & Johnson, "Johnson & Johnson Helping to Reduce Nursing Shortage Enrollment: Rates Up at Nursing Schools Nationwide/More Funding for Nursing Scholarships and Grants," *Johnson & Johnson News*, 2003, *Online*, <http://www.jnj.com/news/jnj_news/20030429_093808.htm>, Oct. 2004.

Johnson, JA; Knudsen, HK; Roman, PM. "Counselor Turnover in Private Facilities," *Frontlines: Linking Alcohol Services Research and Practice,* (Bethesda, MD: NIAAA, 2002).

Join Together Online, "Rewarding Results: Improving the Quality of Treatment for People with Alcohol and Drug Problems: Recommendations from a National Policy Panel," 2003, *Online*, <http://www.jointogether.org/sa/files/pdf/quality.pdf>, March 2005.

Join Together Online, "Hot Issues: Discrimination," 2001, *Online*, <http://www.jointogether.org/sa/issues/hot_issues/discrimination/more/>, Oct. 2004.

Kaplan, L. *Substance Abuse Treatment Workforce Environmental Scan,* (Washington, DC: Abt Associates Inc., 2003).

Keller, DS; Dermatis, H. "Current Status of Professional Training in the Addictions," *Substance Abuse*, 20(3), 1999, 123-140.

Knudsen, HK; Johnson, JA; Roman, PM. "Retaining Counseling Staff at Substance Abuse Treatment Centers: Effects of Management Practices," *Journal of Substance Abuse Treatment*, 24(2), 2003, 129-135.

Knudsen, J; Gabriel, R. *Advancing the Current State of Addictions Treatment: A Regional Needs Assessment of Substance Abuse Treatment Professionals in the Pacific Northwest*, (Portland, OR: RMC Research Corporation, 2003).

Landis, R; Earp, B; Libretto, S. *Report on the State of the Substance Abuse Treatment Workforce in 2002: Priorities and Possibilities*, (Silver Spring, MD: Danya International, Inc., 2002 Draft).

Levin, A. "IOM Report: Building a More Diverse Health Care Workforce," *Health Behavior Information Transfer (HABIT)* 7(2), 2004, Online, <http://www.cfah.org/habit/vol7no2/IOM_report.cfm>, March 2005.

The Lewin Group, Inc., *The Clinical Workforce in the Substance Abuse Treatment System*, (Rockville, MD: DHHS, SAMHSA, 2004).

The Lewin Group, Inc., *Substance Abuse Training Needs Analysis, Final Report*, (Alexandria, VA: The Lewin Group, Inc., 1994).

Mark, T; Coffey, RM; McKusick, D; Harwood, H; King, E; Bouchery, E; Genuardi, J; Vandivort, R; Buck, JA; Dilonardo, J. *National Expenditures for Mental Health Services and Substance Abuse Treatment, 1991-2000*, (Rockville, MD: DHHS, SAMHSA, 2005).

Marks, A. "Jobs Elude Former Drug Addicts," *The Christian Science Monitor*, 2002, *Online*, <http://www.csmonitor.com/2002/0604/p02s02-ussc.html>, Oct. 2004.

McCarty, D. "The Alcohol and Drug Abuse Treatment Workforce," *Frontlines: Linking Alcohol Services Research and Practice*, (Bethesda, MD: NIAAA, 2002).

McLellan, AT; Carise, D; Kleber, H. "Can the National Addictions Treatment Infrastructure Support the Public's Demand for Quality Care?" *Journal of Substance Abuse Treatment*, 25(2), 2003, 117-121.

Meier, PS; Barrowclough, C; Donmall, MC. "The Role of the Therapeutic Alliance in the Treatment of Substance Misuse: A Critical Review of the Literature," *Addictions*, 100(3), 2005, 304 316.

National Association for Addiction Professionals (NAADAC), *The Association for Addiction Professionals' Year Two Final Report: A Survey of Early Career Substance Abuse Counselors*, (Alexandria, VA: NAADAC, 2003).

National Association of Social Workers Practice Research Network (NASW PRN), "Informing Research and Policy Through Social Work Practice," *NASW PRN Survey Final Report,* (Rockville, MD: CSAT, 2001).

National Association of State Alcohol and Drug Abuse Directors (NASADAD), *Recommendations Related to Closing the Treatment Gap,* NASADAD Policy Position Paper, 2003.

National Committee for Quality Assurance (NCQA), "What is HEDIS?" 2005, *Online,* <http://www.ncqa.org/Programs/HEDIS/>, March 2005.

National Committee for Quality Assurance (NCQA), "NCQA Releases HEDIS 2004, 10 New Measures Address Public Health, Service Issues," 2003, *Online,* <http://www.ncqa.org/communications/news/hedis2004.htm>, March 2005.

National Institute on Drug Abuse (NIDA), *NIDA Research Report – Methamphetamine Abuse and Addictions,* (Rockville, MD: NIH, 2002).

National Institute on Drug Abuse (NIDA), *Principles of Drug Addictions Treatment: A Research Based Guide,* (Rockville, MD: NIH, 1999), *Online,* <http://www.drugabuse.gov/PDF/PODAT/PODAT.pdf>, Oct. 2004.

National Survey on Drug Use and Health (NSDUH), *Results from the 2004 National Survey on Drug Use and Health: National Findings,* (Rockville, MD: SAMHSA, 2005).

National Survey on Drug Use and Health (NSDUH), "Nonmedical Use of Prescription Pain Relievers," *The NSDUH Report,* (Rockville, MD: SAMHSA, 2004a), *Online,* <http://oas.samhsa.gov/2k4/pain/pain.htm>, Oct. 2004.

National Survey on Drug Use and Health (NSDUH), *Results from the 2003 National Survey on Drug Use and Health: National Findings,* (Rockville, MD: SAMHSA, 2004b), *Online,* <http://www.oas.samhsa.gov/nhsda/2k3nsduh/2k3Results.htm>, March 2005.

Nevidjon, B; Erickson, J. "The Nursing Shortage: Solutions for the Short and Long Term," *Online Journal of Issues in Nursing,* 2001, *Online,* <http://www.nursingworld.org/ojin/topic14/tpc_4.htm>, June 2004.

New Freedom Commission on Mental Health, *Achieving the Promise: Transforming Mental Health Care in America, Final Report,* (Rockville, MD: DHHS, SAMHSA, 2003).

RMC Research Corporation, "Results of a Statewide Needs Assessment of Substance Abuse Treatment Professionals," *Kentucky Workforce Survey 2002,* (Portland, OR: RMC, 2003).

Rollnick, S; Miller, WR. "What is Motivational Interviewing?" *Behavioral and Cognitive Psychotherapy*, Vol. 23, 1995, 325-334, *Online*, <http://www.motivationalinterview.org/clinical/whatismi.html>, Oct. 2004.

Saitz, R; Mulvey, K; Plough, A. "Physician Unawareness of Serious Substance Abuse," *American Journal of Drug and Alcohol Abuse*, 23(3), 1997, 343-354.

Scanlon, WJ. "Nursing Workforce: Recruitment and Retention of Nurses and Nurse Aides Is a Growing Concern," *GAO testimony*, (Washington, DC: GAO, 2001), *Online*, <http://www.gao.gov/new.items/d01750t.pdf>, Oct. 2004.

Substance Abuse and Mental Health Services Administration (SAMHSA), *A National Review of State Alcohol and Drug Treatment Programs and Certification Standards for Counselors and Prevention Professionals*, (Rockville, MD: DHHS, 2005).

Substance Abuse and Mental Health Services Administration (SAMHSA), *Overview of Findings from the 2003 National Survey on Drug Use and Health*, (Rockville, MD: DHHS, 2004a).

Substance Abuse and Mental Health Services Administration (SAMHSA), *Treatment Episode Data Set (TEDS) Highlights—2002. National Admissions to Substance Abuse Treatment Services*, (Rockville, MD: DHHS, 2004b), *Online*, < http://wwwdasis.samhsa.gov/teds02/2002_teds_highlights.pdf >, March 2005.

Substance Abuse and Mental Health Services Administration (SAMHSA), *The DASIS Report: New Heroin Users Admitted to Substance Abuse Treatment: 1992-2000*, (Rockville, MD: OAS, 2003), *Online*, <http://oas.samhsa.gov/2k3/newHeroinTX/newHeroinTX.cfm>, Oct. 2004.

Substance Abuse and Mental Health Services Administration (SAMHSA), *Trends in Substance Abuse Treatment Admissions: 1992-2000 Treatment Episodes Data Set (TEDS)*, (Rockville, MD: DHHS, 2002), *Online*, <http://wwwdasis.samhsa.gov/teds00/TEDS_2K_Chp2.htm>, Oct. 2004.

Substance Abuse and Mental Health Services Administration/Center for Substance Abuse Treatment (SAMHSA/CSAT), "Addictions Counseling Competencies: The Knowledge, Skills and Attitudes of Professional Practice," *Technical Assistance Publication (TAP) Series 21*, (Rockville, MD: DHHS, 2002).

Taleff, MJ. "The State of Addictions Education Programs: Results of a National Cross-Sectional Survey," *Journal of Teaching in the Addictions*, 2(1), 2003, 59-70.

U.S. Department of Labor, Bureau of Labor Statistics (BLS), *2002-2003 Occupational Outlook Handbook,* (Washington, DC: BLS, 2003).

The Washington Circle Group, "Background of the WC," 2005, *Online,* <http://www.washingtoncircle.org>, March 2005.

The Washington Circle Group, "Specification of Performance Measures for the Identification, Initiation and Engagement of Alcohol and Other Drug Services," (Washington, DC: The Washington Circle, 2004), Online, <http://www.washingtoncircle.org/Final%20Specs%202004_03-30.pdf>, March 2005.

INDEX

#

21st century, 4

A

Abraham, 74
access, viii, 3, 5, 7, 8, 19, 22, 25, 33, 42, 46, 47, 48, 49, 52, 59, 63, 80, 84, 86, 89, 90, 95, 97, 102, 103, 104, 107, 113, 118, 119
accountability, 26, 84, 101, 105, 108, 110, 120
accreditation, ix, 37, 80, 83, 85, 115, 117, 118
administrators, 48, 67
adolescents, 27, 47
adults, 6, 7, 8, 26, 48, 65, 73, 74, 91, 93
advancement(s), 7, 106, 107, 122
African Americans, 11
African-American, 11, 16
age, viii, 8, 14, 15, 46, 79, 89, 91, 111, 112, 113, 116, 124
agencies, 2, 13, 14, 48, 56, 59, 60, 64, 81, 84, 86, 100, 110, 111
aggressive behavior, 93
aging of the workforce, vii, viii, 1
agonist, 97
AIDS, 41, 69, 70, 93, 126
Alaska, 11, 31, 37, 44
Alaska Natives, 31
alcohol abuse, 90
alcohol dependence, 24, 91, 97
alcohol use, 6, 89, 94, 101, 103
alcoholics, 97
alcoholism, 16, 97
ALI, 31
American Psychiatric Association, 39, 40, 41
American Psychological Association, 40, 41
antidepressants, 25
antisocial behavior, 43, 93
anxiety, 94
anxiety disorder, 94
APA, 112
Appropriations Committee, 2
assessment, 13, 25, 37, 45, 57, 72, 75
assets, 87
asthma, 98
attitudes, 97, 117
authorities, 50, 51, 64, 118
autonomy, 109, 120
avoidance, 104
awareness, 9, 28, 33, 67, 95

B

ban, 103
barriers, 6, 14, 16, 26, 32, 39, 100, 113, 116

base, 13, 16, 23, 26, 27, 28, 29, 30, 33, 36, 37, 38, 39, 40, 41, 46, 47, 48, 49, 50, 55, 70, 81, 86, 95, 96, 108, 116
behavioral disorders, 19
behaviors, 100
benefits, 57, 67, 74, 90, 101, 103, 105, 110, 122
blood, 8, 93
blood pressure, 8, 93
blood vessels, 93
bonuses, 78, 120
brain, 93
brain damage, 93
breakdown, 10
budget line, 33
Bureau of Labor Statistics, 3, 10, 15, 18, 20, 21, 110, 132
burn, 13, 16
business management, 110

C

caliber, 116
cancer, 71
candidates, 20
care model, 8, 25
career development, 61
caregivers, 69
Caribbean, 28
CDC, 93, 126
Census, 11, 77, 128
certification, 10, 11, 14, 19, 21, 23, 25, 29, 32, 42, 74, 78, 81, 86, 112, 117, 118, 123
CFR, 57
challenges, vii, viii, 1, 2, 4, 19, 25, 27, 39, 42, 46, 80, 81, 84, 85, 86, 87, 88, 95, 101, 105, 107, 119, 122, 123, 125
changing environment, 105
chemical, 19
Chicago, 67
child abuse, 73
child development, 46
childhood, 46
children, 5, 27, 42, 43, 46, 47, 65
cholesterol, 96, 97

city(s), 48, 76, 126
classroom, 46, 71
classroom environment, 46
clients, 19, 43, 84, 86, 92, 93, 96, 98, 107, 111, 113, 115, 118, 124
clinical presentation, 92
coaches, 25, 32, 43, 54
cocaine, 91
collaboration, 2, 25, 31, 33, 43, 44, 48, 60, 66, 68, 70, 71, 98, 110
collateral, 35
college students, 45
colleges, 29, 45, 63, 116, 119
commercial, 92
Committees on Appropriations, viii, 80
communication, 10, 30, 113
community(s), 3, 10, 13, 16, 19, 20, 22, 26, 28, 30, 34, 36, 42, 45, 46, 47, 48, 49, 50, 51, 52, 53, 54, 55, 56, 57, 60, 61, 62, 63, 65, 66, 67, 69, 74, 95, 96, 99, 100
community service, 48
community-based services, 48
compensation, vii, viii, 1, 2, 6, 12, 15, 17, 21, 22, 79, 84, 87, 122, 123
competitive grant program, 63
compilation, 57, 58, 75
complement, 115
complexity, 101, 111
compliance, 51
composition, 6, 24, 118
compounds, 108
computer, 71, 107
computer technology, 107
conference, 33, 60, 70
confidentiality, 57
confrontation, 95
Congress, v, vii, 1, 4, 19, 76, 79, 86
Congressional Budget Office, 24, 72
consensus, 27, 85
consent, 57
consumers, 27, 54, 62, 66
contingency, 95
continuous data, 61
control group, 99
controlled substances, 70

Index

conviction, 103, 104
cooperative agreements, 45
coordination, 46, 60
correlation, 125
cost, 7, 8, 19, 23, 37, 77, 90, 102, 120
cost benefits, 90
cost of living, 120
counsel, 44
counseling, 19, 41, 52, 68, 74, 87, 107, 117, 121
counterbalance, 15
creativity, 109, 120
credentials, 106, 112
criminal justice system, 103
critical thinking, 6
culture, 3, 5, 115
curricula, 30, 36, 40, 41, 48, 65, 66, 69, 71, 83, 115, 117, 118
curriculum, 32, 36, 41, 48, 54, 55, 59, 63, 67, 69, 71, 116, 117, 118, 119
curriculum development, 59, 67, 117, 119

D

data analysis, 53
data collection, 14, 27, 28, 58, 61, 62, 102
data set, 3, 29, 58
database, 50, 58, 59, 78
deaths, 8, 44
deficiencies, 6, 84
demographic characteristics, 123
demographic data, vii, 1
dental care, 66
Department of Health and Human Services, viii, 2, 80, 126
Department of Labor, 2, 10, 15, 18, 20, 21, 60, 71, 120, 121, 132
depression, 8, 9, 24, 52, 78, 93
detection, 101
detoxification, 97
diabetes, 9, 71, 82, 98
diet, 96
directors, 13, 14, 16, 20, 21, 28, 29, 43, 108, 116
disability, 23, 41, 123

discomfort, 23
discrimination, 10, 15, 51, 103, 104, 128
diseases, 9, 94
disorder, vii, 1, 2, 6, 7, 19, 24, 26, 29, 30, 36, 52, 92, 94, 95, 96, 99, 100, 102, 104, 105, 111, 115, 117, 120, 121
dissatisfaction, 90, 106
distance education, 66
distance learning, 33
distress, 24
distribution, vii, viii, 1, 12, 22
District of Columbia, 28, 41
diversification, 105
diversity, 34, 62, 69, 74, 85, 101, 111, 113, 119
doctors, 114
domestic violence, 9
drug abuse, 4, 30, 90
drug addict, 16
drug addiction, 16
Drug Enforcement Administration (DEA), 92, 93, 127
drug interaction, 38
drug treatment, 75, 106, 125
drugs, 43, 70, 92, 93, 101, 103

E

earnings, 90, 120
educational attainment, 8
educational experience, 39
educational institutions, 83, 111, 113
educational materials, 30, 40
educational practices, 119
educational programs, 118
educators, 9, 10, 24, 25, 38, 46, 54, 62, 63, 71, 118
elders, 69
elementary school, 46, 113
e-mail, 38, 107
emergency, 36, 43, 69, 92, 100
emergency preparedness, 69
emotional disabilities, 49
emotional exhaustion, 13, 74
emotional health, 78

employees, 75, 120
employers, 104
employment, 10, 19, 26, 40, 57, 74, 81, 86, 102, 103
empowerment, 7
enrollment, 63, 113, 116
environment(s), 28, 46, 53, 57, 87, 98, 105, 109, 118, 120
equity, 3
ethics, 41
ethnic background, 22, 66, 111, 113
ethnic minority, 22, 34, 35, 118
ethnicity, 124
evidence, 4, 5, 6, 8, 13, 23, 24, 25, 26, 27, 28, 30, 33, 36, 37, 38, 42, 45, 46, 47, 50, 60, 62, 66, 73, 85, 87, 92, 94, 95, 98, 102, 105, 108, 115, 116, 119, 122
evidence-based practices, 4, 5, 6, 8, 13, 24, 25, 27, 60, 62, 66, 73, 102, 108, 115, 119
evidence-based program, 46
examinations, 117, 118
execution, 28
exercise, 96
expenditures, 94, 104
expertise, 43, 59, 105, 116
exposure, 34, 93

F

faith, 28, 81, 86
families, 3, 5, 46, 53, 59, 63
family income, 24
family members, 28, 62, 63, 114
family therapy, 112
fast food, 17
FDA, 97
federal agency, 2
federal government, 42
fidelity, 27
financial, 8, 51, 67, 103, 120, 122
financial incentives, 103, 120, 122
financial resources, 8
flexibility, 25
focus groups, 16, 75
food, 17

Food and Drug Administration, 97
force, 23, 44, 45, 63
formal education, 16, 39, 115
funding, ix, 2, 3, 14, 20, 23, 26, 28, 32, 33, 34, 36, 38, 39, 40, 41, 42, 44, 45, 47, 48, 51, 53, 54, 58, 60, 63, 64, 65, 68, 80, 89, 94, 95, 101, 104, 110
funds, 28, 29, 36, 38, 42, 45, 50, 51, 58, 59, 60, 100, 103

G

GAO, 121, 131
general knowledge, 34
general practitioner, 121
Georgia, 119
good behavior, 8
graduate education, 40
grant programs, 63
grants, 19, 34, 35, 53, 54, 65, 67, 69, 70, 71
growth, 3, 21, 24, 27, 62, 93, 111, 120
growth rate, 21
guidance, 84
guidelines, 39, 49, 58, 70
Gulf Coast, 13, 14, 16, 21, 73

H

Hawaii, 44
Health and Human Services, viii, 2, 80, 126
health care costs, 5, 104
health care professionals, 22, 36, 83, 111
health care system, 66, 71, 85, 103, 111, 116, 122
health condition, vii, 1, 8, 24, 26, 34, 54, 78
health education, 115
health information, 5, 20, 26, 70
health insurance, 5, 24, 63, 123
health practitioners, 5, 53, 63, 72
health problems, 8, 49, 55, 69, 78, 93
health promotion, 71, 73
health services, 4, 6, 7, 14, 23, 24, 25, 34, 49, 52, 62, 70, 75, 83, 95, 100, 112, 119, 120

Index

heart disease, 82
heart rate, 93
hepatitis, 70, 93, 97
hepatitis c, 70
heroin, 69, 90, 92
HHS, viii, 2, 24, 31, 60, 72, 76, 77, 80, 126
high blood pressure, 8
high school, 12, 113
high school diploma, 12
higher education, 115, 118
hiring, 67, 97
history, 16, 28, 87
HIV, 41, 69, 70, 97, 126
HIV/AIDS, 41, 69, 70, 126
homelessness, 91
homes, 24, 55
hospitalization, 10
host, 20, 70
House, viii, 57, 66, 80
housing, 10, 102, 103
human, viii, 75, 79, 81, 83, 86, 109, 115, 116, 123
human resources, 109
Hunter, 73
hypertension, 97, 98

I

identification, 9, 63, 122
identity, viii, 72, 80, 85, 105
illicit drug, viii, 6, 24, 43, 79, 89, 93
image(s), 114
immersion, 32
improvements, 7, 85
in transition, 118
incidence, 93
income, 14, 19, 22, 24, 120
Indians, 31
industry(s), 17, 19, 107
information sharing, 53
information technology, 5, 20, 26, 82, 84, 107
infrastructure, viii, ix, 3, 38, 74, 79, 80, 85, 87, 90, 95, 102, 103, 105, 106, 107
ingredients, 22

initiation, 102
institutions, 33, 68, 83, 111, 112, 113, 117, 118, 119, 122, 125
integration, 3, 5, 6, 7, 9, 24, 25, 26, 49, 54, 55, 60, 64, 65
internship, 53, 61, 62, 65
intervention, 4, 26, 36, 42, 45, 47, 95, 100, 104
investment(s), 52, 87
Ireland, 73
issues, vii, viii, 1, 2, 3, 4, 5, 11, 13, 21, 23, 26, 27, 31, 34, 39, 41, 42, 46, 53, 58, 59, 60, 61, 62, 63, 64, 69, 79, 81, 84, 85, 87, 88, 89, 90, 101, 104, 108, 109, 111, 121, 123, 125, 128

J

job performance, 109
job satisfaction, 120
juvenile justice, 9, 47

L

landscape, 3
Latinos, 50
laws, 3
lead, 2, 8, 45, 55, 59, 86, 92, 93, 94, 113, 123
leadership, ix, 31, 33, 34, 44, 47, 66, 80, 82, 108, 109, 110, 121, 122
leadership development, 31
learning, 33, 47, 48, 51, 66, 71, 107, 112, 118, 119, 122
learning process, 47
legislation, 3, 7, 64, 72
level of education, 29, 84, 124
lifetime, 94, 103
light, 24, 51
local community, 26, 46
logistics, 47
longitudinal study, 73

M

magnitude, 101
majority, 4, 17, 20, 22, 26, 29, 45, 85, 95, 100, 102, 115
management, ix, 10, 17, 32, 37, 45, 51, 55, 59, 67, 71, 74, 80, 82, 89, 95, 97, 98, 99, 100, 105, 107, 108, 109, 110, 120, 121
marijuana, 91, 92
Marine Corps, 81
marketing, 35, 73, 83, 113, 121
marriage, ix, 11, 34, 53, 68, 80, 81, 85, 86
materials, 9, 30, 35, 38, 40, 43, 44, 58, 60, 70, 116
matter, 59
measurement, 101
media, 111, 113, 114
median, 13, 14, 17, 19, 78, 90, 120
Medicaid, 4, 8, 19, 24, 32, 51, 58, 63, 73, 77, 81, 99
medical, 8, 20, 36, 37, 38, 41, 44, 47, 52, 66, 67, 69, 90, 91, 92, 93, 97, 98, 99, 103, 109, 111, 112, 114, 116, 120
medical care, 8, 97
Medicare, 81
medication, 9, 10, 25, 26, 70, 97, 99, 105
medicine, 36, 56, 66, 83, 100, 111
membership, 16, 50
mental health professionals, 22, 40, 41, 66
mental illness, vii, viii, 2, 3, 4, 7, 8, 12, 15, 16, 20, 23, 24, 26, 31, 40, 48, 53, 54, 55, 57, 63, 72, 75, 78, 93
mental retardation, 20, 66
mentoring, 32, 33, 37, 38, 39, 110, 122
mentorship, 120
messages, 113
meta-analysis, 13
methadone, 37, 97, 98, 111
Methamphetamine, 130
methodology, 123
mid-career, 16
military, 3, 5, 37, 65
minorities, 11, 20, 34, 113, 116, 118
minority students, 118
mission, 3, 87

Missouri, 76
misunderstanding, 15, 16
misuse, 38, 83, 122
models, 13, 23, 25, 30, 43, 54, 55, 63, 98, 99, 123
modules, 70
momentum, ix, 80
mood disorder, 94
morale, 121
morbidity, 38
mortality, 38, 72, 75
MR, 127
MSW, 18

N

narcotic, 81
National Child Traumatic Stress Network, 47
National Health Service, 52, 57, 65, 126
national policy, 102
National Strategy, 44
National Survey, 6, 76, 77, 89, 93, 126, 128, 130, 131
next generation, 67
Northern Ireland, 73
ntac, 77
nurses, ix, 16, 26, 34, 37, 40, 43, 67, 68, 80, 81, 83, 84, 85, 86, 97, 98, 106, 111, 112, 114, 115, 116, 119, 121
nursing, 65, 66, 98, 113, 114, 121

O

OAS, 131
obesity, 8, 9
ob-gyn, 100
Office of National Drug Control Policy, 57, 66
ONDCP, 65
operations, 56, 119
opioids, 37, 38, 39, 69
opportunities, 13, 24, 33, 34, 39, 44, 49, 50, 51, 57, 60, 68, 85, 105, 106, 107

oral surgeon, 37, 67
organizational culture, 101
organize, 66
OSHA, 70
outpatient, 14, 74
outreach, ix, 50, 68, 80, 85, 99
overlap, 88
oversight, 59

P

Pacific, 11, 28, 127, 129
pain, 37, 38, 39, 67, 69, 91, 97, 130
pain management, 37, 67, 97
parity, 3, 4, 7
parole, 19, 48
participants, 16, 31, 40, 41, 47, 50, 54, 55, 99
pathways, 61, 68
patient care, 8, 84, 121
peer review, 118
peer support, 32, 55, 57, 70, 72, 99
per capita income, 14
performance measurement, 101
permit, 102, 111, 117
personal responsibility, 10
pharmaceutical, 97
pharmacology, 37
Philadelphia, 13
physical health, 8, 26, 102
physicians, ix, 9, 13, 14, 24, 25, 26, 36, 37, 38, 55, 66, 67, 69, 71, 80, 81, 83, 84, 85, 86, 97, 98, 106, 111, 112, 115, 116
pipeline, 61, 67, 68
platform, 85
PM, 128, 129
police, 48
policy, 30, 31, 32, 42, 49, 51, 101, 102
policy makers, 101
policymakers, 46
pools, 107, 113
population, vii, 1, 4, 5, 6, 8, 11, 12, 21, 23, 38, 63, 84, 85, 89, 92, 93, 101, 104, 111, 118
portfolio, 51

positive relationship, 17
poverty, 24
prejudice, 6, 12, 16, 25, 51
premature death, 90
preparation, 26
preparedness, 69
prescription drug abuse, 4
prevention, vii, 1, 4, 5, 8, 9, 23, 31, 32, 34, 39, 40, 43, 44, 46, 50, 52, 56, 63, 78, 123
primacy, 8
principles, 27, 39, 99, 113
private sector, 20, 101
probation officers, 19, 48
professional development, viii, 29, 79, 84, 87, 106, 107, 109, 123
professionalization, 32
profit, 16, 78, 100
programming, 32, 64, 67
project, 3, 28, 30, 32, 37, 43, 48, 49, 59
promote innovation, 5
protection, 61
psychiatry, 36, 41, 42, 43, 66
psychological distress, 24
psychological health, 5
psychology, 53, 65
psychosocial interventions, 97
psychotropic medications, 25, 97
PTSD, 5, 9
public awareness, 9
public education, 55
public expenditures, 94
public financing, 81, 88
public health, 5, 8, 9, 23, 25, 39, 94, 111, 121
public policy, 101
public sector, 42, 95, 102, 120
public service, 17
publishing, 35
Puerto Rico, 28
pulmonary diseases, 9
purity, 92

Q

qualifications, 14, 21

quality improvement, 5, 6, 7, 85, 102, 103
quality of life, 96
questionnaire, 59

R

race, 10, 124
racial minorities, 11
RE, 127
recognition, 22, 36, 80, 103, 106, 114, 116, 120
recommendations, viii, 4, 58, 62, 71, 80, 81, 82, 85, 86, 88, 105, 106, 109, 111, 116, 122, 125
recovery, viii, ix, 5, 7, 8, 9, 22, 25, 27, 28, 29, 31, 32, 40, 47, 49, 62, 63, 71, 72, 78, 79, 80, 81, 82, 84, 85, 86, 87, 89, 99, 100, 104, 105, 106, 109, 114, 122, 124, 125
recovery process, 25, 87, 99
recruiting, 4, 13, 14, 16, 20, 21, 27, 29, 59, 90, 98, 110, 122
reform, 3, 5, 7, 9, 64, 103, 126
Registry, 127
regulations, 57, 70
rehabilitation, 10, 66
reinforcement, 95
relevance, 116
remission, 99
requirements, 17, 19, 20, 51, 63, 87, 98, 101, 118
researchers, 30, 81, 86, 101
Residential, 20
resilience, 87
resistance, 95
resources, 2, 4, 5, 8, 30, 31, 32, 33, 39, 47, 49, 52, 56, 58, 60, 77, 87, 89, 90, 95, 101, 109
response, viii, 29, 80, 96
retardation, 20, 66
retention rate, 119
retirement, 63
revenue, 17, 89
rewards, 22, 120
rings, 111

risk(s), 5, 8, 9, 23, 27, 36, 37, 43, 44, 45, 55, 56, 94, 95, 96, 98, 100, 122
risk assessment, 37, 45
risk factors, 55
rowing, 92
rules, 85, 95
rural areas, 14, 27, 65, 108
rural population, 68

S

safety, 48, 61, 62
savings, 8
scarcity, 7, 64
school, 12, 33, 43, 46, 53, 66, 100, 113, 115, 118, 121
science, 26, 27, 30, 39, 50, 63, 85
scientific knowledge, 87
scope, 22, 123
self-image, 114
Senate, viii, 2, 80, 120
serum, 97
service provider, 44, 47, 48, 101, 120
short supply, 22
shortage, 14, 22, 42, 86, 105, 114
showing, 90
signs, 55
skills training, 95
smoking, 8
snorted, 93
social activities, 10
social consequences, 90
social identity, 72
social relations, 8
social relationships, 8
Social Security, 41
Social Security Disability Insurance, 41
social services, 19
social skills, 95
social skills training, 95
social support, 13
social workers, vii, ix, 1, 11, 14, 19, 21, 24, 26, 34, 36, 40, 41, 43, 52, 53, 55, 65, 68, 80, 81, 83, 85, 86, 106, 112, 115, 116, 117, 121

society, vii, viii, 2, 16, 19, 95, 98
solution, 113
SP, 127
specialists, 8, 9, 10, 12, 22, 23, 24, 25, 32, 38, 40, 53, 65, 66, 99, 101
specialization, 105
spending, 28, 94
Spring, 129
SSI, 41
stability, 102, 120
staff development, 84, 95
staffing, 11, 45, 98, 101, 105, 107, 110
stakeholder groups, 81, 86
stakeholders, viii, 5, 28, 49, 52, 58, 60, 64, 80, 84, 86, 105, 106, 109, 110, 116, 123, 125
standardization, 23
state(s), 4, 10, 12, 15, 17, 19, 23, 24, 25, 28, 29, 30, 32, 34, 39, 41, 42, 44, 45, 46, 48, 49, 56, 58, 61, 63, 71, 75, 98
statistics, 67
stigma, viii, 2, 79, 83, 84, 86, 104, 114
stimulant, 91
strategic planning, 64, 110, 122
stress, 13, 19
stroke, 93
structure, 106, 107, 117, 122
subscribers, 31
subsistence, 120
Substance Abuse and Mental Health Services Administration (SAMHSA), vii, 2, 64, 72, 77, 131
substance use disorder(s), viii, 6, 7, 8, 9, 15, 25, 26, 28, 29, 31, 35, 48, 70, 79, 90, 91, 94, 95, 96, 98, 99, 101, 102, 115, 116, 117
suicide, 4, 42, 43, 44, 45, 56, 94
suicide attempts, 45, 94
summer program, 67
supervision, 5, 13, 27, 29, 42, 62, 63, 71, 74, 108, 109, 115, 120, 121
supervisors, 13, 30, 81, 82, 86, 108, 109, 123
support services, viii, ix, 49, 72, 79, 80, 109
Supreme Court, 24, 72

sustainability, 108
symptoms, 8
synthesis, 58
systemic change, 36

T

TAP, 117, 131
target, 35, 38, 101, 113, 123
target population(s), 38, 101
Task Force, 44
TBI, 5
teachers, 43, 46, 119
teams, 8, 13, 24, 27, 56, 62, 63, 98
technical assistance, 5, 28, 40, 41, 43, 44, 47, 48, 49, 50, 53, 54, 57, 58, 59, 67, 82, 102, 107
techniques, 30, 37, 95
technology(s), 4, 5, 6, 20, 26, 30, 36, 61, 62, 63, 70, 82, 84, 90, 101, 103, 107, 108, 109
technology transfer, 4, 30, 82, 90, 103, 108, 109
telephone, 28
testing, 41, 42
therapeutic communities, 74
therapeutic relationship, 12
therapy, 38, 97, 107, 112
thoughts, 44, 45
tobacco, 71
tracks, 33, 50, 102
trade, 71, 81, 86, 122, 125
trafficking, 127
trainees, 41, 53, 72
training programs, 36, 62, 71
transformation, 40
translation, 56
trauma, 5, 9, 36, 47, 48, 49, 65, 77, 100
treatment facility, viii, 80
treatment systems, viii, 79, 89, 104
trial, 48
tuberculosis, 97
turnover, vii, viii, 1, 2, 11, 12, 13, 17, 21, 23, 39, 71, 73, 74, 75, 84, 90, 101, 106, 108, 109, 110, 119, 120

U

U.S. Department of Labor, 120, 121, 132
uniform, 117
uninsured, 19, 24
United, 7, 11, 13, 21, 22, 63, 72, 76, 77, 103, 117, 120, 126, 127
United States, 7, 11, 13, 21, 22, 63, 76, 77, 103, 117, 120, 126, 127
universities, 29, 45, 115, 116, 119
urban, 22
urban areas, 22
Urban Institute, 127
USA, 17

V

variables, 22, 78
vessels, 93
victims, 65
videos, 35
violence, 9, 47, 77
vocational rehabilitation, 10
Volunteers, 127

W

wages, 17, 18, 19, 39, 110
waiver, 67
Washington, 44, 73, 74, 101, 102, 126, 127, 128, 131, 132
web, 29, 33, 39, 40, 44, 70
websites, 37
welfare, 9, 46, 75, 90, 91, 100, 103
welfare reform, 103
welfare system, 91
wellness, 10, 46, 57, 63, 66, 122, 123
White House, 57, 66
work environment, 109, 120
worker shortages, vii, viii, 1, 2, 12, 13, 84
working conditions, 110
workplace, 115

Y

yield, 123
young people, 113, 114